vanishing shoals

vanishing shoals

a memoir

First published in 2022 by
Life in 10 Minutes Press
Richmond, VA

lifein10minutes.com/press

Distributed by IngramSpark
& Life in 10 Minutes Press

ISBN 978-1-949246-19-3

Printed in the United States of America

First Printing, 2022

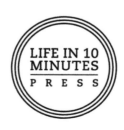

vanishing shoals

a memoir

Sita Romero

Issue 7 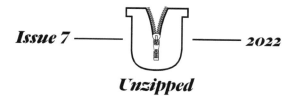 2022

Unzipped

Shoal²
/SHōl/

a sandbank or sandbar that makes the water shallow;

a hidden danger or difficulty

Praise for *Vanishing Shoals*

In *Vanishing Shoals*, Sita Romero takes the reader with her on a journey—not just of a cancer diagnosis and treatment, but of youth and grit, parenthood and divorce, hardship and friendship, and the lessons in all of it, the graces and gifts. Romero reminds us that it's the people who truly love us that keep us afloat and who will save us until we know how to save ourselves. *Vanishing Shoals* is a journey of fear and doubt, hope and spirit. Romero doesn't offer pat answers or easy endings, just as life doesn't: we humans—at our best—take one step and then another, understanding the risks, willing ourselves to go out into life's depths and move forward through it anyway. Romero does just that.

— Shuly Xóchitl Cawood, author of *The Going and Goodbye: a memoir*

Romero's writing perfectly captures the endless ebb and flow between grief and salvation. As a narrator, Romero expertly drops readers into the moment of devastation—a cancer diagnosis—then rewinds the clock to her childhood where we meet a girl gaining familiarity with loss, sickness, and the quivering thread that tethers us to mortality. *Vanishing Shoals* is the story of a hard-won victory, the struggles that predated, and the after-fight that never truly ends.

— Samantha Otto Brown, Author of *Sub Wife: A Memoir from the Homefront*

Switching from the past to the present, Romero creates beauty out of disaster. Readers will find much to relate to in this memoir of a difficult and confusing childhood, and the way it impacts the journey to healing from a terrifying cancer diagnosis.
— Gabi Coatsworth, Author of *Love's Journey Home*

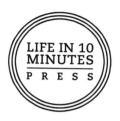

About *Life in 10 Minutes*

Life in 10 Minutes is a community of writers sharing stories that are brave and true through classes, workshops, retreats, Zoom, and our online lit mag. Visit **lifein10minutes.com** to read deep, strange, hilarious, heartbreaking, and powerful stories written 10 minutes at a time, and share yours, too!

Homegrown in Richmond, Virginia, *Life in 10 Minutes Press* began with the mission to give passage to books we believe in. We seek to bring readers titles that are brave, beautiful, raw, heartfelt, and vital, and to nurture authors in their publishing journeys.

Learn more at **lifein10minutes.com/press**.

Our mission: We are especially passionate about memoir by women and under-represented voices, nonfiction that challenges the status quo, and boundary-breaking books of all genres. All works published with Life in 10 Minutes Press *are carefully chosen to support our mission and reflect our commitment to promoting fresh, engaging, high-quality storytelling.*

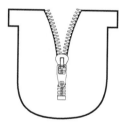

Welcome to *Unzipped*

Life in 10 Minutes fosters love of the immediate. Of the present. The truth. As close up as we can possibly get. At *Life in 10 Minutes*, we reveal life in this moment, right here, right now. Feelings and memories rise from our bodies and spill onto the page. Our stories have curled into knots in our stomachs, fists squeezed around our hearts, pressure against our lungs. We allow these stories to unfurl in our notebooks, releasing us from their grip. As we write, we heal ourselves. As we share our stories, we heal each other. As we heal each other, we heal the world.

Never before has healing the world felt more urgent than now. Now, when connection is more tenuous and precious than ever. When truth is on the chopping block. When the world is on literal and metaphorical fire, when unhealed family and systemic and global trauma threatens to pull us into our most base and destructive selves.

Writing and sharing and reading our stories allows us to process the past, ground in the present and move into the future, freer and more deeply woven into the life-giving, rich fabric of human life. When we write unzipped, we reveal the naked truth, the vulnerable core. When we write unzipped, we join a community of other writers who agree to hold each other's stories and bear witness, to listen, to believe. To create space for the sacred and profane to exist together on the page.

Punctuation is not our first priority. You might find minor errors. You might see a mistake on the page. Sometimes the writing will reflect the chaotic messiness of urgency. We decided that getting the work out there was more important than getting everything perfect.

***

When we opened a call for submissions in the fall of 2021, we could only dream of receiving a manuscript as vivid and skillfully rendered as Sita's. We were as thrilled with our very first reading as we are now, presenting Sita's micro-memoir to you. In *Vanishing Shoals,* Sita Romero vacillates between the chilling story of what it's like to grow up with a narcissistic, addict mother and what it's like to deal with aggressive cancer as an adult mother. The language sways from haunting to humorous, from objective to full-on in-the-moment sit-in-it emotion. She carefully leads you between the safe spaces within the scientific language of -omas, the nonverbal cues between cancer patients, the breaking points between mothers and daughters, and the role of forgiveness in unforgivable situations.

***

Stay tuned for *Unzipped* Issue 8, a memoir by Slats Toole. Slats "feels most at home in liminal spaces, in the spaces between, in the both/and, in paradox, contradiction, and tremor" and proposed the memoir to us as exploring "my narrative not as logical movements from point A to point B, but as what is created in the space between my different, often seemingly contradictory, experiences and paths. I hope to release myself and the readers from the expectation of life looking a certain way, allowing us to make meaning through whatever experiences we have."

With love,
Dr. Cindy Cunningham and Valley Haggard, Co-Editors
Llewellyn Hensley, Graphic Designer
Nadia Bukach, Director of Operations

Looking for a past (or future) issue of *Unzipped?*

If you missed past issues, they are available for order on the *Unzipped* website (**lifein1ominutes.com/unzipped**).

Issue 1, *Wild Woman: Memoir in Pieces,* by Cindy Cunningham,

Issue 2, *She Lives Here,* by Kristina Hamlett,

Issue 3, *Unraveled Intimacies,* Paula Gillison, Lisa Loving, Mary Jo McLauglin, Sema Wray,

Issue 4, *Inheritance,* by David Gerson and Stephen McMaster,

Issue 5, *There's No Accounting for the Strangeness of Things,* by Valley Haggard,

Issue 6, *Bare: An Unzipped Anthology,* edited by Cindy Cunningham and Valley Haggard

— *Life in 10 Minutes Press*

About Life in 10 Minutes Press

About the press:
Homegrown in Richmond, VA, *Life in 10 Minutes Press* seeks to give passage to brave, beautiful, raw, heartfelt, and vital works as we nurture writers in their publishing journey.

Learn more at *lifein10minutes.com/press.*

Mission: We are especially passionate about memoir by women and under-represented voices, nonfiction that challenges the status quo, and boundary-breaking books of all genres. All works published with Life in 10 Minutes Press are chosen carefully to support our mission and reflect our commitment to promoting fresh, engaging, high-quality storytelling.

We are infinitely grateful to our patrons who make it possible for us to continue publishing urgent, brave, and true stories. Subscription is the best way to support our mission, and helps us cover the costs associated with producing our quarterly publication.

To subscribe, visit **www.lifein10minutes.com/unzipped.**

vanishing shoals
a memoir

Author's Notes

The work of a memoir is always, and should only be, seen as one person's account. I am sure there are other versions of some of these stories. There are certainly other perspectives. It is with honest sincerity that I offer these musings as my own, the way that I remember them. Any mistakes are mine. There are fuzzy moments from the past and even the present. You will find that I dabble in maybes and perhapses. There are some moments that are crystal clear. There are remembrances and there are gaps filled in with my own imagination or coping. I have not given the actual names of all my teachers or some of the fellow students, but the people themselves are real. I have done my best, limited by the nature of memory and minds. My goal was never to write with objective authority, but rather to explore with subjective curiosity. Nothing is ever all of one thing. During my time working through my rare cancer diagnosis, I had an honest experience of weighing life and death. Through that exploration, I uncovered some truths about my spirituality, upbringing, and my own tenacity.

It was not my goal to write a cancer memoir. It was my goal to take down the details of that year—the moments, the feelings, and the events with a precision that would allow me to understand them later. I had no idea it would turn into anything more than a diary for myself. The stories of my past bubbled up during my year with cancer, demanding my attention. Only after the experience began to fade did I connect the dots and put all these pieces together, weaving something bigger than my spirituality, my cancer, and my childhood.

"Everybody I know who wades deep enough into memory's waters drowns a little."

— Mary Karr

Dedication

For Marcos, who always believed it would only be a chapter.

Acknowledgments

This micro memoir would not have become what it is without the people who have been part of this journey with me.

Thank you Whitney, for sending me the submission call and believing that my story was something L10 press would be interested in. But more than that, thank you for showing up big for cancer, for laughing at it with me, for crying with me, and for braving it all the way. Your humanity, deep insight, and long conversations helped me bring some of these thoughts to the page. You will see yourself in here as a crystal quartz, carried with me into chemotherapy. You will recognize some of your own words of wisdom.

Thank you to Donna, Whitney, and Densie for reading early, messy first drafts and helping me shape the individual pieces.

Thank you to Shuly for welcoming me into a memoir writing class during treatment when I knew that what I was going through would be a story to tell one day. You helped me find my CNF voice, but more importantly, you helped me find the guts to share it.

Thank you Katie, Kelly and Cheryl for helping me remember details from the past that have become fuzzy and unclear. I never would have recalled the name of that Video store on my own.

Thank you Brandee, Kiana, Marcos and Tracy for participating in the Namestorm Brainstorm and sharing your insights in an attempt to name this work. I know I can be finicky about titles and had a hard time landing on this one. Thank you Rogue Writers, Lita, Gabi, Lisa and Stephanie, for spending half the session on me that week and coming at the memoir sideways with your title ideas.

Thank you to the team at L10 press, Valley, Cindy, Nadia, and Llewellyn for all the behind the scenes work, the multiple read throughs and the attention to detail. Thank you for believing in me and seeing that this was a story that should be told.

Thank you to my ARC readers, Sam, Gabi, Shuly, Kiana, Brandee, Ayla, and Jenn. Thank you for the kind praise, words of encouragement, and gift of your time.

Thank you to my therapist at MSK, Kimarie, who allowed me to see the truth of my story—that I am allowed to take, without guilt, all that I have learned from my parents and use those skills throughout my life. And that the gifts they gave me are mine to own, hold and use. Thank you to my other therapists, Sandy and Carly, for book-ending my cancer year with your insights.

Thank you to my head and neck cancer support group who was there for all the gory details of cancer and life from 2020 and beyond, most especially, my SNUC buddy, Dave. It meant the world to me to walk this journey with someone else living in a patient's skin. Thank you for seeing the glow in my eyes when my new skin grew back, complimenting my eyebrows, and reminding me regularly about meeting dates.

Thank you to the women who walked their cancer journeys before me, sharing bravely, talking me through comfort measures, and being open about your own journeys. Jennifer, Lora, Autumn and Barb, you helped me find the nerve to share.

Thank you to my family of origin. I want you to know that I am healing and I wish you well.

Thank you to my in-laws for raising such an emotionally intelligent human whose upbringing around sickness and health allowed him to take it all in stride. Thank you for taking in our youngest children as your own so I could fight the fight with everything I had.

Thank you to my children for your strength in the face of this diagnosis, for holding each other through hard moments, for braving the time apart, and for continuing to grow into your best selves, not letting cancer derail you from your truths. Stand tall and let the world see you for who you are. I'm so incredibly proud of you all.

Most of all, thank you to my amazing husband, Marcos, who lived through this experience with me. Thank you for being present for all the nitty gritty: the crying, the head shaving, the sickness, the driving, the feeding, the moving, and more emotional support than I ever thought husbands capable. It's okay that you let me hit the floor that one time, you caught me eventually. Thank you for being my Perrin, for a love so deep you would burn the whole world to keep it. Every day I wake up and honor the rareness of this kind of love.

The News That Changed Everything

September 2020

You are about to hear news that is going to change your world. The doctor is going to point at the gray spot on your MRI and tell you why she thought it might be an encephalocele at first. You will turn to your husband and tell him, "That's not what they think it is anymore," before the doctor gets to the punchline.

You will look around the room and wonder why no one told you to sit down to receive the information. You will think of the TV shows and movies you've seen where the characters sit down for their bad news.

Your brain is not going to be able to process it all at once, although it will try. You will immediately have thoughts about your mortality, your children, your husband. You will feel guilt and terror and it will shift rapidly to gratitude that you found the tumor and you will tell your husband that you can brave it because you would be so much worse in his shoes.

You will have to start making phone calls to deliver the news. You will not remember to tell people to sit down. You will cry when you hear your friends crying and you will think of how horrible it must feel to receive the call. Watching life unfold while you live in it doesn't stop you from trying to see the story from everyone else's eyes.

You will worry about dumb shit in the days leading up to the "official" diagnosis. Things like your eyebrows, what to wear when you leave the house during the pandemic, and how others might judge you once your hair falls out.

You will worry about bigger things too. Like the cost of cancer, how your kids are expected to cope through this big, scary thing, and your already overactive nervous system handling the extra anxiety of cancer.

You will tell a friend, "If I die, I need you to help my book live out in the world." You will tell your husband, "If I die, I need you to be everything to our children in my absence." You will tell your doctor, "I think it's time I start on anxiety meds," knowing you have needed them for years.

You will wonder what you did to "get cancer," like it's something you could have planned for or controlled. You will question food you ate and products you put on your skin. You will ask the universe how you earned this karma. You will want to control things that are outside of your control. You will clean up your diet, meditate, and join a support group where you are the youngest person in attendance.

You will get a second opinion. You won't even want to go to the consult, but you trust your husband with your life, and you know he has gently and lovingly guided you in the right direction. You will take your kids to stay with friends and move to New York City so you can be treated by someone who has seen this cancer before.

You don't know how the story ends. You want to write it like a piece of fiction with a satisfying story arc. But real life is messy. Complicated. Unpredictable. Instead, you make a promise you hope to keep—to live through it, to allow it to be part of your story, and to find the voice to share it.

The California Ashram

1983

The grass tickles my skin, but I spread out in it, luxuriating in the morning sun. The temperature is neither hot nor cool; it is the perfect spring weather that entices everyone out onto the lawn.

I flick the blades of grass and rub my palm along the greenery, tickling my hands over and over until they become used to the feel of the gentle caress. There is a picnic blanket and food, but I can't be bothered with that when there is so much to see and do.

My older brother is there, fuzzy in the memory, but present, his ginger hair shining in the morning light. The little one is not yet conceived. Mother wears her hair long to her waist, parted in the center. She is fresh faced, her oversized glasses taking up space and covering the dark chocolate beauty mark on her left cheek. To me, she is vintage, from a magazine in the seventies.

Dad can't sit still. He plays with my brother, laughing. His hands itch for his guitar, longing to make music. He stands and walks in silent meditation, taking in the family he has created.

A blond woman with Farrah Fawcett hair comes over and speaks to Mother. She compliments the beautiful children, as if we are set pieces in the play my parents are enacting. They speak quietly while I turn my body into an oblong rock and roll down the hill, letting the grass envelop me. I know it will itch later, but I do it anyway.

I make my way back and my mother turns to me, smiling, and brushes me briskly. She doesn't chastise me for getting my clothes dirty. She doesn't ask me not to roll again. She doesn't tell me to sit or to be quiet.

When the women finish their conversation, each of them forms their hands into prayer, nods, and whispers a farewell greeting. It is a mantra, a sign of reverence, a hello, a goodbye. Like aloha, it has more than a single meaning.

Years later, I describe the place to my mother. I want to go back there. I want to live on the hill where the sun shone, where we lived a happy, shiny life. I want to play in the space where my parents were quiet and reverent. I want to sit in the warm sun and bask in the gentle breeze.

She is shocked that I recall the hill. But she recovers quickly and reveals that the hill is on the opposite coast. It is outside the Ashram in California where my parents lived when I was born. We are settled now in the east. It holds its place in my mind as my earliest memory. She tells me I was only three and assures me that the memory of my toddlerhood is real. But what she doesn't say is also real. That life is gone.

Between the Eyes
October 2020

"We found a sinonasal mass." I nodded and wrote the words in the top of my notebook, as if I were a secretary taking down notes. I barely comprehended what it meant.

She pointed at a spot on the fuzzy black and white image on her computer screen. I could make out the orbits of the eyes, the familiar skeletal image. My husband held my shoulder from behind. I scribbled more notes, trying to capture what she said so I could absorb it later.

Between the eyes.

Blocking the smell nerves.

Tumor.

"But there's no way to know exactly what it is with this imaging," she said.

"How will we know exactly what it is?"

Biopsy.

I needed to sit.

The nearest chair held her laptop bag and a purse or maybe her lunch. She'd brought us into her office to look at the images on her computer. I thought that if it were my office, my bags would be there too. I stumbled around the desk and dropped into a chair.

My brain processed too fast and simultaneously moved in slow motion.

I looked up at Marcos, his face serious and serene, even with a face mask blocking his nose and mouth. "Do you need to sit?"

He shook his head. "No. I'm good." I looked at the other chair, but it was too far away. Even if he needed it, he wouldn't have taken a chair across the room.

I put the pen back to the page. "What are the possibilities? What could it be?" I had to focus. I had to ask questions, even if I didn't really want the answers. Even if I couldn't understand them yet.

"Let me write them for you." She pulled her own strip of paper from her desk and started writing.

The long, slender sticky pad said "Work Hard" at the top and had a colorful chicken in the bottom corner.

Work hard.

Melanoma.

Sarcoma.

Lymphoma.

Why are all the -omas settled there between my eyes?

Esthesioneuroblastoma.

Sinonasal endocrine carcinoma.

Sinonasal undifferentiated carcinoma.

Oma. Oma. Oma. Is that word supposed to mean something? *Tumor. It means tumor. And Grandmother?* My mind shifted to my grandmother who died of lung cancer. I think of my father going up to be with her at the end. We arrived at the funeral days later where I saw my cousins for the first time in years. I wanted to look at the last picture of her, wearing a wig to mimic her natural hair.

Chondroma. The last possibility preceded the chicken on the sticky pad, but he ran toward it with bright yellow, red, blue, and purple plumage. I couldn't look away.

She wanted me to go to Johns Hopkins in Baltimore, three hours north of home.

"They are the best," she said.

I read a book about the research they'd done there—research conducted on the poor in a time when research was compensation for treatment. And now I am sent because of insurance and accessibility and my own privilege. Was that supposed to be a blessing?

I cried off and on.

I nodded.

I asked more questions.

It couldn't be real.

I stood.

It was over. Or maybe it was just beginning.

I looked into the doctor's eyes and saw that they were red and watery. She had let her humanity in and allowed herself to sympathy cry with me. I imagined how she probably usually holds it in. I thought about how she has a fence built around her emotions, caging them. But they'd spilled over and in that moment, I felt seen and understood. I witnessed her being a woman and a human—so much more than a doctor delivering bad news.

I could only think to thank her. "Thank you. Thank you for being human and handling this with such care and grace. You are remarkable and I know this is the worst part of your job."

I had the sense that she might have hugged me if we hadn't been keeping six feet of social distance in the new COVID-world. She stood behind her desk in her mask, and I stood with Marcos, holding him, clutching my little blue book of bad news. I left her office with a world of knowledge I didn't want.

In the car, I told Marcos we could sit for a bit and talk if he wasn't ready to drive. How could he get the news that his wife has a giant tumor in her face and then drive off? How could he stay between the lines, use his turn signal, and pretend that our world wasn't crumbling?

The office assistant came out of the front door directly to our car. I wondered if I forgot something inside. I masked my face again and opened the window.

I stared, mesmerized by her bedazzled mask glittering in the light. "I just want to tell you I'm praying for you. My thoughts are with you and your family."

I nodded and thanked her, numb.

That would be my new normal. People telling me how their prayers are with me and my family.

I wanted to tell her it might not be that bad.

It might be ok.

I needed to say it or at least think it.

Even if I wasn't sure if I believed it.

Drowning
1985

A skinny man in blue shorts responded first to the high-pitched scream. My shoulders tensed. I clutched the Barbie doll, her wet hair dripping over my hand like the ice cream in my other. The skinny man in blue shorts dove into the pool, his body knife-like, arms out front, ankles together. Sharp, focused, intent. An Olympic-worthy dive.

It wasn't until he surfaced with the baby in his arms that I realized why the woman in the sleek bikini had been screaming. A white linen dress pooled at the woman's feet. Maybe she was undressing to go in after the baby? Maybe her scream was enough to summon whoever's job it was to rescue drowning babies?

My baby brother's face, though reddish purple, remained angelic. He was a beautiful blond-haired boy. Tears ran down his cheeks, mingling with the chlorinated water. I dropped the doll and the ice cream.

My mother came running, shock and hysteria apparent on her face. The skinny man held my baby brother up from the side of the pool and my mother bent and scooped him up, clutching him to her body. Her own tears matched his, despite her effort to calm him.

I stood and swiped at my bottom, brushing the flecks of dirt, wiping at the pilling fabric of my worn swimsuit.

My father appeared, red-faced. He glared at my mother, his eyes accusing. It would not be a quiet ride home. Tonight would produce noises long into the night.

I left the poolside after a half-hug with my pig-tailed friend to change into my dry clothes before the ride home; the suit clung to me like a second skin.

We said goodbye to the hosts, making our way out of the crowd. After the quiet moments filled only with my brother's cries, the partygoers had gone back to their beers and chatter. My baby brother had calmed. He sat in his carseat sucking on the corner of a blanket, the wadded, wet cloth in his mouth. My older brother and I slid in beside him.

My mother furiously whispered to my father outside of the car, thinking the closed doors provided a barrier of privacy. They stood on the driver's side as she tried to wrestle something from his hands, her face a storm of emotions. He had thick sausage-like fingers, but he looked clumsy, and she yanked too hard, the silver gleamed against the summer sky as the keys flew into the grass. A look of determination in her eyes, she turned as if she might dive into the grass like a baseball player sliding into home. My father threw his hands up and stomped to the other side of the car. I turned to see Mrs. West in the doorway shaking her head beyond the shadow of the screen door.

My mother slid into the driver's seat. My father plopped into the passenger seat and slammed the door. Yes, the change of drivers meant tonight would be a yelling night. A fight night.

It would be a night when my mother would burst into my room, there to use my eyes and ears as armor against violence. Mom's bruises told a story. The gaping cut on Dad's side and broken ceramic pieces of a dinner plate in the trash told another. But for now, we were safe and dry, and my brother had been rescued from the pool, and that was worth something.

Orphan

November 2020

"Are you going to die?" our sixth grader asked.

Once the words were out, all thoughts that came before and after seemed muted and insignificant.

Our youngest child has always been tall for her age. When she was only three, the daughter of a family friend, at age seven, complained to her mom because everyone wasn't helping clean up toys post-playdate. Her mother gently reminded the girl that the red-headed wild child was only three years old, but she refused to believe it. Adding to the problem is how articulate she's been next to same-age peers. She likes to talk, express ideas, and share opinions. But when she gets tired, she can melt down just like any other child.

She's also always been a "sensitive" person. It's not a term I love, but to me, it means she feels things deeply and can often articulate those deep feelings. When she is at a loss for words, the deep feelings come out in her behaviors. She nursed the longest, slept in our bed the longest, and regularly gets away with being the youngest of four. Although she stopped making nightly appearances in our king-size bed by the age of three, any nighttime disturbance, nightmare or whim can bring her back into our bed in the middle of the night. She will slink stealthily beneath the covers, careful not to wake us, so that she will not be walked back to her own bedroom. In the morning, we'll find her sleeping peacefully between us, her long lashes fluttering through her REM sleep and the spray of freckles across her cheeks prominent in the morning sunlight.

We shouldn't have been surprised by her words. She is intelligent, emotionally and otherwise, sensitive and brave. But when she crawled into our bed, nearly six feet tall at age eleven, and began to cry, her words shook us to our cores.

I had already called the pediatrician. "Do you have any resources for supporting children through their parent's cancer diagnosis?" They were stumped and passed me over to the American Cancer Society. I read through their helpful tips.

I approached my best friends about the topic, and collected their advice, filing it away for the moment when I might need it. *Be honest. Don't overpromise. Reassure. Only share what is age-appropriate. Hold back your own fears and worries.*

"Are you going to die?" is not a yes or no question, in most ways. Of course I am going to die, because we are all going to die. But that was not really her question. Are you going to *die from cancer?* Are you going to die *soon* is what she meant with her question. Part of me wanted to answer with a joke: *I have never told you this before, but I am not immortal. Sorry to disappoint.* But through her sobs, I knew she needed a real answer. She needed the truth. Don't overpromise. What would I want to hear if I were the one asking this question?

I steadied my voice and did the best I could. "I don't know what's going to happen. But I can promise you this: I will fight this with every fiber of my being. We are going to go wherever we have to go and be treated by the best of the best. I will endure whatever it takes to fight this cancer. And I can also promise you this: you are strong and no matter what happens, you will survive this."

She wanted to hear that I would survive it. But what if I didn't? We'd done the research on this rare sinus cancer. The numbers weren't good. The doctors all told us: *Stay off the internet. Maybe don't even specify the type of cancer with your friends and family. They will Google and it will scare them.* This cancer used to be a death sentence. The chance of survival was not favorable before the doctors at MD Anderson discovered a new way to treat it. About 40% of people beat it. Then a new study published in 2019, the year before my diagnosis, posited a treatment option that offered an 80-90% cure rate, if the patient responded to the initial treatment plan.

We had contemplated going to MD Anderson for treatment. Clearly, they were literally writing the book on this cancer treatment. It was all so new, and our doctors at Hopkins were excited to set me on the path of the new protocol and watch to see if my body responded. Responding to the initial chemotherapy became the key to predicting individual outcomes. But it was information we were months away from at that time. I hadn't even begun the first treatment yet. I had a head full of hair, a heart full of hope, and my arms were full of my youngest child, curled in a ball in my lap, crying about my potential exit from this world.

My words did not comfort her. "But we are in a pandemic. What if dad catches COVID and dies? I'll be an orphan if you die too."

She had probably been worrying about her father's demise since the beginning of the pandemic. We were in unprecedented times, pre-vaccine, locked down from the outside world. She had stopped going to in-person school, stopped seeing friends, and wore a mask on the rare occasions she left the house. Food and necessities were delivered to our door. The world had become a dangerous place and now I faced a serious diagnosis—and I couldn't promise I was going to live through it.

She wailed in my arms as we offered comfort to her. I recited the words from the American Cancer Society. I recited words from my best friends, in search of anything short of a false promise. Marcos added to what I said, holding firm in his belief that we would beat it. His unshakable faith strengthened me. "Your mother is a strong woman. And so are you. We can all be strong now for her as she goes through this. I know it's scary."

Comfort. Validate. Don't overpromise.

Children shouldn't have to worry that Death is coming to their doorstep. They should not have to live trapped in a fantasy, orphaned, imagining life without two parents. Where would she live? Who would raise her? How long would it hurt? When would she know for sure if I would live or die? If she should mourn or move on?

She stayed in our bed that night, cuddled between us, snug under the covers in a place of safety, her feet reaching the foot of the bed, her long arm draped over me, secure in the thought that I was there, right now, real, and in her arms.

Summer in the Catskills
1988

The ashram's welcome center, open and bright, reminded me of the kind of swanky resorts I'd seen in commercials, but instead of vacationers, it was crowded with swamis dressed in orange robes.

Once we were checked in, our family of five made our way to our apartment—a small one-room studio with a private bathroom I was surprised we could afford. We lived in Sadhana Katir, the most "affordable" option of the dorms. Only women and children stayed on our floor, maybe even in our whole building. Mom assured me that we would all do *seva*, service to the guru, to support the cost of the trip.

That summer, my brothers and I spent several hours each day in the woods at the Children's House, where I met my best friend for the season. Chaitanya—who we called Cai—had bronze skin and dark brown curls. His lashes, long and curled like his hair, made his eyes look a bit feminine. He climbed trees, played hide and seek, and thought up magical stories with me. The director of the children's program encouraged us to make art, always focused around the Guru and her teachings.

A playful joy surrounded Cai, a contagious happiness. His eyes lit up with excitement at climbing, running, and playing. His art had bold colors, the strokes bravely committed to his page. When the director announced a children's play, Cai shone as one of the leads, playing a deity adorned in shining embroidered silks. Cast as a swaying tree, I stood happily in the corner for my role.

When we'd left home for our summer in the ashram, I hadn't known that my parents were on the verge of a divorce. I just knew we had been given the opportunity to be with the Guru, and we were taking it. Dad drove us up to the Catskill Mountains in South Fallsburg, New York. The farthest we'd ever traveled had been from our home in Florida to my grandparents' house in Georgia. I had just finished third grade.

I saw Washington, DC out the window, the Washington Monument visible above the skyline from the highway. We didn't have the time or money to add tourism to our trip. But pressing my face to the window and watching the gleaming white buildings stream by felt like a gift. We stopped for gas in Philadelphia and an elderly Black man approached the window with a dirty rag. My mother shooed him off, as if he were one of the oversized Florida horseflies that bit me every summer. He pretended not to see her and cleaned the window.

"That was nice of him," I said.

"No," she said. "It's a trick. He cleans it first and then expects you to pay him."

I rolled the idea over in my head. It wasn't the first time I'd heard the message loud and clear—the world was a tricky place. People were out to get you and didn't have your best interest at heart. It would not be the last time I heard it.

When the Catskill Mountains came into view, it appeared with a presence unlike anything I'd seen in flat Florida. We'd been transported to a magical place. My ears clogged with the altitude change and Dad taught us how to pop them by swallowing. I swelled with pride, anticipation, and wonder viewing the tops of trees crowded on the slopes in the mountains.

Beyond the drive, I have no memories of my father from that summer. I don't know how long he stayed after delivering us to the Hudson Valley ashram. We just knew he had to get back to Florida and back to work. Though he'd left the Air Force after only a short stint, that experience plus two years of college landed him a job in civil service that did not allow for three months leave.

Our daily routine began the next morning. Meals were eaten in the dining hall, Guru Gita in the morning, playing at the children's house, seva, intensives, evening talks, chanting, and meditation. The regularity comforted me. There were no surprise shouting matches, quiet accusations or anyone "falling asleep" on the living room floor. No one blasted Zeppelin to drown the noise of life, and no one played guitar with a far off look in his eye. The only music came in the form of chanting.

We ate breakfast, lunch, and dinner with the other residents in a large cafeteria. Devotees doing seva served the meals and Mom reminded us to eat whatever was presented and be thankful. I don't remember feeling hungry at all that summer or wondering what we might scrounge up for a meal, nor did I ever throw any of my food away, no matter how strange it seemed to me. I had already been vegetarian my whole life and Dad regularly cooked Indian food on Sundays. Many of the dishes were familiar and I quietly swallowed the rest.

In the evenings, we chanted in the great hall for hours. Sometimes, I would lay my head in my mother's lap or put my cheek to the carpet when I became too tired to stay seated in my cross-legged position. We listened to Gurumayi give talks multiple times each week. With an inviting smile, warm golden flawless skin, and a square jaw, she was the most beautiful person I'd ever seen. She entered the room like I imagined a queen might, commanding the attention of the audience, dressed in orange from head to toe. "I welcome you all with all my heart." An aura of humility surrounded her. The greeting became a mantra, the familiar sentence offered to us each time, and I felt her heart opening to the whole room. Mom spoke of the Guru's importance, of how she sat at the side of her own Guru for years until he was ready to *leave his body* and pass his position to her. Even at eight years old, I felt pride and empowerment that our Guru was a woman.

None of the women at the ashram wore makeup. Everyone dressed in modest clothing. Both men and women wore flowing linens and cotton pants that hung loosely from their bodies. People walked in silent meditation, mala beads moving through their fingers as they prayed. Other women called my mother Jayashree, her spiritual name, instead of her given name. She had taken on the persona of a devotee—chanting, meditating and pretending that the characters we played at the ashram were the same as in our real lives.

I received Shaktipat that summer, an awakening of my Kundalini energy. The intensive, led by an older white swami, replaced the week's regularly scheduled events, which were canceled in favor of our "turn" at the next level of spiritual practice, study, and devotion. I didn't know exactly what it meant, but I accepted my spiritual awakening as a rite of passage, blessed by the guru, who showed up at the end of the week to grant us the honor.

It would awaken our inner spirits. It would enable us to be more devoted, more dedicated, and it would deepen our meditation practices.

At night, the four of us slept in the single room. I shared the larger bed with my mother, and the two boys slept side by side on another mattress on the floor. We never fought bedtime because the morning devotion would come early before the sun. Sleeping in or "being lazy," as my mother put it, was never an option. Satsang, seva, or meditation beckoned us seven days a week.

One afternoon, mom dropped me off in one of the many meditation rooms located on campus. I don't remember if she needed me to be occupied because she had something to do, or if I had misbehaved and therefore sent to meditate as a punishment. It wasn't the great hall where we meditated as a group, but a small building near our living quarters.

Even as a child, I took myself seriously. Time to meditate meant serious concentration and nothing else. In a hushed whisper, she reminded me to behave as I opened the exterior door to the darkness of the muted room.

With an older brother barely more than a year my senior, I had become used to being a younger sibling, a shadow to him. That day, dropped off alone, I felt proud that I could be responsible enough to be left by myself. My friend, Cai, already sat in meditation when I arrived, but the room otherwise remained empty. I found a spot next to Cai and settled into position. We didn't play, or open our eyes and peek at each other, or crawl around the floor. We curled our legs into the best Lotus position we could manage, we sat with our backs ramrod straight, and we said our mantras silently over and over.

So'Hum. I am.

I saw the curved line between the words in my mind, like a sideways parenthesis that connected the two words and between them, a raindrop in my mind's eye. My breathing slowed. Time slowed. I watched the raindrop, the curve, the mantra. It came easily to my serious, focused mind. It had been practiced enough times that a familiar peace settled over me.

Later, when my mother came to pick me up, she ushered me out of the room hurriedly, her energy opposite from my relaxed state. A bit dazed from the quiet, dark room and the concentration of my meditation, I blinked into the sun, registering panic on her face.

"Where did you go?" she asked me.

"What do you mean, where did I go? This is where I went...and you brought me here." Why didn't she know that?

"But you stayed in there the whole time?"

I looked at her, confused. "Yes. That's what I was supposed to do, right?"

"Well, yes, But I guess I didn't know you would do it for so long."

I blinked again. "How long has it been?"

"A long time."

I shrugged.

She relaxed. "Did you have a nice meditation?"

Now I smiled, proud of myself. "Yes, and my friend Cai was there, but we didn't play."

Her eyes narrowed. "Did you sit close to him?"

"Yes. Why?"

She took my hand and walked me back to our little apartment at Sadhana Katir. "It's just that you want to keep your energy separate from others. You didn't touch him when you meditated, did you?"

I thought of my hand grazing his when we formed our mudras on our knees. Yes, I had certainly grazed his hand. It had been dark in there, and I'd been comforted by my friend who'd come to meditate, although he hadn't stayed nearly as long as I had. But I could tell what my answer should be. "No," I said. "But why?"

She let out an audible sigh. "Cai has a brain tumor, you know. He is here to try to clear out that negative energy."

A sadness settled on me. I knew without her saying that Cai was not likely to live into adulthood. But he didn't seem like a sad kid. He had been a beautiful Lord in the play. He ran and laughed and played just like everyone else our age. I don't remember doing anything kind for his family. My mother didn't hold his mother's hand as she cried over her child's diagnosis. I never got an address to send letters after the summer ended.

The biggest part of his illness, to me, had been in that singular moment when my mother revealed it, sharing his secret. I wasn't sure if I was supposed to acknowledge it with him or pretend I didn't know. She had shared the news so matter-of-factly that I felt shame for my sadness. She talked about his diagnosis being his karma, somehow earned from another lifetime, here to follow him and haunt him. It was his problem, and not ours, from her perspective.

The biggest takeaway Mom wanted me to have was that I should not touch him, as if his brain tumor might energetically leave his body and enter mine.

Cancer Class

November 2020

I haven't been in the classroom since I graduated from my MFA program. But my cancer diagnosis came with a flurry of new information. I'd started taking notes with a small blue spiral-bound journal in my ENT's office. Then I graduated to a full-size composition book, and then onto a binder to house all of my appointment notes, doctors, medications, dates, phone numbers, symptoms and the list of people to send thank you notes.

My cancer binder has a label on the front. It says Fuck Cancer.

My Type-A organizational Self could not have been happier to find out that day one of Chemotherapy came with a class. One way to quiet my Anxiety Brain is to give it information. My Anxiety and I went to class and sat in the front row, ready to take notes and earn that gold star. To my delight, I received another Binder, this time with more tabs and less profanity.

While the internet may be a plethora of information, even more would be gained in the class.

Every cancer treatment is different, and individuals respond differently to treatment. No promises that you will survive.

Call Oncology if you have any questions or concerns. Can they answer this one: Why is this happening to me?

There is a protocol for chemo-tainted bodily fluids. I'm going to be "contaminated" for 48 hours after treatment.

No French kissing or hot sex for 48 hours. Do people have sex after chemo?

Close the lid and flush twice, with preferably no one else sharing the bathroom. So my husband and I should not share the bathroom? I am to send him and his bad kidneys somewhere else?

In the event of a night sweat, change the contaminated sheets (with gloves). This reminds me of changing sheets soggy from leaky diapers.

No raw meats or fish. No sushi?

No crowds. The pandemic already addressed this one.

No guests who are sick. No guests at all.

Everyone washes hands upon entering the house from any ventures to the outside world. Ventures to the outside world include: The wig shop, doctor's appointments, treatment, and the pharmacy.

There are resources: This includes social workers, psychologists, nutritionists and even alternative therapies such as acupuncture. Be prepared for this treatment to fuck up more than your hair.

Unfortunately, there were no gold stars at the end of class. I decided to write an A+ on the first page of my binder.

From the Spiritual Gift Shop

2020

When the box arrived, I swept it off the porch and stashed it before anyone could see who had sent it. It had been seven years since I'd spoken to my mother.

It didn't come from my mother's Florida address. The label had the name of the ashram and a Pennsylvania address. It was addressed in my mother's name with my home address. When I brought the box in and showed my husband, he said, "Obviously it's from her." Once I'd smuggled it up to my bedroom in private, I stashed it in my closet, waiting for the moment I might feel ready.

The day before we began the three-hour drive to Baltimore, I started a suitcase with everything we might need. I began with essentials— the cancer binder, the gallon-sized Ziploc filled with prescriptions to address the multitude of side effects—medications for anxiety, nausea, pain, and more. The list would grow throughout treatment, but the cancer starter-kit consisted of more medication than I'd ever taken in my life. I packed the new pajamas and socks which had been delivered in a care package. I still had my hair, so I packed hair ties and comfortable clothing and sweaters. I gathered extra items for my new tote deemed the "chemo bag" that I would soon take with me on my eight-hour solo journey through my first infusion. It had been lovingly curated by a friend with a swear-words coloring book and mindfulness journal. It held lip balm, a battery pack, a book, my laptop, and the start of a knitting project. She'd also included a heavy, clear quartz crystal that hid tucked into the inside pocket. In my mind, that crystal was my friend there with me at chemo. I may have to go in there physically alone, but I knew she would be with me. As I held the crystal, I thought of the box stashed in my closet.

I paused during packing, removed the box from the Spiritual gift shop from the closet, opened it, and unpacked each item one by one. I found a book with full-page quotes from the Guru and a card with a picture of Her. I wondered at how she'd aged over the years because her Guru headshot looked the same as it had been on our altar since the eighties. I uncovered a CD, but I lacked a CD player. The largest item of all unfolded as a deep royal blue cashmere-silk meditation shawl embroidered with the sacred Om. I fingered the tassels and thought of the shawls I'd seen on my mother through the ashram years. Last, I found a message stone engraved in both English and Sanskrit.

I dug for a note, wondering what words could close a seven-year gap.

All I found was a packing slip nestled in with the gifts. It itemized the content, but did not include a personal massage.

I palmed the smooth stone, a polished lapis lazuli disrupted only by the single word—Prashānti.

Shānti, a word I knew to mean peace. Prashānti, Peacefulness of the Self. I tucked the cool marbled stone in beside the crystal, and packed the shawl into my suitcase. Maybe it wasn't possible to heal the wound between us. But I would bring her with me to chemo, the token of her tucked in between the folds of cloth. I stashed the rest of the box in my closet, unsure what to do with the relics from a religion long abandoned. But before filing it away, I nestled the image of the Guru between the pages of my current book.

The next morning, we loaded the car. Dogs, kids, snacks, my favorite pillow, and suitcases piled into our car for the trip.

The COVID pandemic resulted in restricted access to the cancer center. It had been made very clear that I would go alone. There were not yet vaccines approved even for emergency use and a ward filled with compromised immune systems meant no support people physically present. The weight of it crushed Marcos, but he held a brave face.

"I would love for you to be there and hold my hand. But the kids need you. I can do this. I know I can handle it." I forced the words, wanting to believe them. In the end, it would be my fight. I had plenty of supporters all around me. But when it came time to face the monster, I had to do it alone. No one could do it for me. No one could take it from me, no matter how hard they wanted to.

As I stood in the driveway while we loaded the car, my eyes fell on Dad's boxes. The haste of his departure from his time living in our home had resulted in boxes-worth of belongings left behind. I had moved them three times since his coma, to storage, and then amongst my own things, bringing them along when I left the state and settled in Virginia. They were heavy with poetry, statues of the Buddha, sacred jewelry, linen shawls, newspaper clippings, old letters, and the remnants of his altar, which used to be meticulously adorned in the small bedroom he had claimed for his coma recovery.

I called my dad frantically. We had only spoken once since my diagnosis. Our conversations usually tally to two per year. I said the words fast, rushing them out. "I know I still have a lot of things of yours in boxes here. I know you wanted them back. But now I have to go to my first chemo and...is there something in your boxes you want me to take with me?"

"You are welcome to anything in my boxes. Help yourself."

I had wanted him to tell me what to take. What was the most spiritual? What was the most important? He had taken the sacred tulsi beads to my grandmother as she died of lung cancer. She left this world with his religious relic around her neck and his guitar music in her ears. It reminded me of the beads we'd all worn as children. There must be a sacred mala, blessed by someone. I wasn't sure if any of those things meant anything to me. But it had meant something to my father, and a piece of my mother lay nestled inside my chemo bag, so it only seemed appropriate.

In the end, I settled on a singular rudraksha bead, the thick brown leftover of a dried stonefruit, believed to carry a high energy and safeguard the wearer from negative energies. For good measure, I also put on Dad's tulsi necklace, thought to purify the body, mind, and spirit and help the wearer overcome health issues.

Both of my parents came with me to chemo. They weren't there. They never saw me bald or brought me ginger ale when I puked. They never dropped off dinner or took the kids for ice cream. They never did things that parents might do when their grown child has cancer. But they were with me, in the room, when I took on the chemo treatment.

Sometimes, I sank into my mantras from childhood. I could hear my mother's voice from back then, "say Om Namah Shivaya," she'd encourage as she poured hydrogen peroxide to clean a scrape on my knee. I'd squeeze my eyes shut and repeat the familiar words over and over. Now, the mantra lives in my mind, like a nursery rhyme recalled with rote memory. When the nurse started my IV, digging to find the right vein, I thought, "Is this when I repeat Om Namah Shivaya over and over?" The old raindrop would appear at times when I sat in the infusion chair. The raindrop and the curve. *So'Hum.*

Sometimes, I avoided my old mantras completely. I turned to a guided meditation for chemotherapy, visualized myself on the beach surrounded by everyone who supported me, coming to cheer me on for treatment. I saw a long-haired man with a beard on that beach, standing next to the fountain of life, connecting me to the pouring water and energy the way my IV connected me to the chemo drugs. Maybe it was my husband, dressed in white with an angelic face. Maybe it was Jesus. Maybe it was both, or something my subconscious mind fabricated completely. Whoever he was, he had a presence in the room, ensuring that the chemicals pouring from my IV were joining my body in an effort to heal, not harm.

I guess some people find God when they have to look Death in the face. I found my childhood, uncovered it from the rubble in my brain and leaned gently toward it.

Riptide

1989

I learned to take the ocean for granted. It happened gradually, but it's inevitable when you grow up close to the beach. In Florida, the beach isn't just for summertime. It's warm nine months out of the year.

Other families went to church on Sundays. Some girls put on their best Sunday dress and shiny Mary Janes and I put on my swimsuit and sunscreen. We worshiped at the altar of the ocean and listened to the gospel of the waves.

Dad convened with the ocean as if it were his God. He never rested on the sand like a sunbather. Instead, he swam with us, taking us out beyond the breakers, past the foam into the calm buoyancy where we might lose touch with the sea floor momentarily when the wave swept us up. We learned to flip onto our backs and float, meditating with the rhythm of the Atlantic.

Dad sat with us in the sand, building sandcastles, complete with turrets and sand peaks, built drop by drop. We walked along the shore, skipping in and out of the surf, slowing by the washed-up shells to search among them for shark's teeth. On cooler days, we'd find sand flea colonies by chasing the v-shape and bubbles and digging the tiny crustaceans out of their shoreline burrow. If we got bored of any of those activities, we'd grab the paddles and rubber ball and play paletas. Most of the time, the beach exhausted us and we had to beg Dad to take us home. If money allowed that week, we were gifted sub sandwiches to eat on the ride home. I can still feel the cool air blasting in the sub shop. The smell of the shop right after the beach is seared into my memory.

Sometimes, there were lifeguards watching from their oversized orange wooden chairs. But before Memorial Day or after Labor Day, beachgoers, including us, were on their own. But we knew to watch the flags.

Green. Yellow. Red.

One Sunday before their divorce, Mom took us to the beach by herself for the first time. I don't know how the negotiation happened behind the scenes. Maybe he told her, "I can't be there this Sunday, but the kids still want to go. Please take them." Maybe it had been another fight for the books. And he won. Maybe he didn't ask her to take us, but we asked, begging her not to break our Sunday tradition because he was out of town or whatever the case had been that day.

We piled in the car, sweating without air conditioning, then shivering because the highway blew the wind so furiously. Since Mom drove and Dad wasn't there to take up the last remaining seat in our five-seater car, I brought a new friend to the beach. They'd just moved to Florida and she'd never seen the ocean before. My oldest brother sat up front, taking the spot that would forever become his after Dad left, and my little brother squished into the back with me and my friend.

It started like most other Sundays. We searched for sand fleas. We played paletas. My brothers and I took my friend out to swim. The sandbar created a divider in the ocean. The shallows, tidal pools, and ankle-deep water provided a spot for games. Half-submerged, we crawled around, pretending to be mermaids or sea creatures. The sandbar privilege belonged to the older kids. My big brother, my friend, and I got to venture out of the shallows, leaving my little brother behind.

A new game ensued. Maybe we were pirates or lost merpeople, and when we reached the sandbar it became our home base—a castle only we could see. We had graduated from the tidepools, but were not beyond the breakers since Dad wasn't there. We were neither at the shore, nor were we deep in the ocean, but somewhere in-between. Our own private island.

The tide turned. The waves crashed at us into the sandbar. Then the water rose quickly enough to sweep grown adults off their feet and drag them out to sea. The rip current pulled and the merpeople lost their castle. The sandbar vanished beneath our feet, the current roughing it away and we were deep in the water, in a place I used to think of as safe. The familiar salty seawater washed over me. I went under. I wanted to push off the sandy bottom like I kicked off the side of the pool to push myself farther, propelling my way back to shore. But I couldn't find the sandy bottom. My brother yanked me back to the surface.

"I'm tired. I can't swim back."

The shore in the distance appeared farther than I had ever seen it. I pushed against the current, trying to make my way back toward the beach, but no matter how hard I kicked and pulled, it wasn't getting any closer.

On the sand, my mother lay quietly in the sun, her eyes closed. She had never been the play-in-the-ocean parent. She did not accompany us on shark-tooth searches or castle builds. She watched us from the blanket as she baked in the sun. But on this particular day, she had gotten high, and the warmth of the sun called her to the blanket, where she lay flat. Asleep.

When she tells the story later, crying, she will say, "The Guru came in the form of that woman, and she tapped me. She said, 'Are those your kids?' As she woke me up, I stood, and screamed for help."

Three men ran into the surf, plunged into the water, and swam for us. I remember holding onto the shoulders of a burly guy and asking, "Can you touch yet?" He didn't want to tell me no, so he gave me an evasive answer and I thought, *I am smart enough to know that means no.*

A strong swimmer, he was the merperson that I was not. He swam for the shoreline with me on his back, as I tried not to choke his neck in my fright. After a while, I pestered him again, like we were on a long car ride together. *Are we there yet?* But I posed the same question, "Can you touch *now?*" I didn't fully exhale or stop asking until he finally said yes. Yes, he can touch. *Yes, we will survive. Yes, you are safe.*

Afterwards, I sat between the dunes, huddled with my family (minus Dad), crying. We sheltered in the shade of the dune hill, embraced by the warm, fluffy sand. My little brother cried, too. He didn't understand why, but we were all upset and so he sensed the mood and joined us as small children do. I cried because I thought I might not make it back. I cried because I had become too tired to swim. I cried from the fear that had risen inside me. What if I had given up? I cried in relief that my big brother had yanked me back up.

My friend cried. Later, when she told her mother about her beach experience, her mother did not believe her.

But the tears I didn't understand were my mother's. She had not been the one choking on salty water. She had been sleeping peacefully on the beach. Yet her hysteria howled above ours, louder than the rest of us. Her immediate telling about the Guru (in the form of a Florida beach-goer) saving us from the rip current, came through between her sobs.

On the drive home I kept thinking, *Dad will never trust you to take us by yourself again.*

Beam On

January 2021

"Does it hurt?" I asked.

"No, you can't even feel it."

"How long is the radiation?"

"Total time is about 15 minutes but the radiation itself is only a couple of minutes."

Every day. For thirty-five days.

While the nurse said I might not have any mouth or throat symptoms since the tumor is at the skull base, the doctor reminded me about the lymph node treatment in my neck, which would likely result in disturbing the lining and impacting my swallowing ability. I collected each new piece of information, gathered and stored it, increasing (or, less often, decreasing) my anxiety.

Once the radiation therapist took me, she gave me instructions to gown up and I waited in a pretty room with a fireplace loop on the television. I got to keep my pants, so my legs stayed warm as I waited in the thin gown.

The therapists introduced themselves and showed me the machine. I settled on the metal table, lying in a foam molded for my unique shape. They brought me a blanket that stayed warm for thirty seconds, but the weight on my body and the act of a blanket for comfort seemed right.

They strapped the mask on, a device I would wear daily that locked me to the table. It fit tighter than I remembered from the simulation. I tried to tell them, mumbling through the bite-piece. The therapist yanked the hardened plastic, creating a slight adjustment but there just wasn't much to give. It pressed heavily on the right side of my forehead and pulled on my upper left teeth. But I thought about how it would only be a few minutes so I gave the thumbs up.

First, the table wheeled itself 90 degrees and positioned me beneath the machine. I expected it to move all around me based on their explanation, the table remaining stationary. There were always two radiation therapists, and that day, one had a heavy accent. She told me they'd take two images first and then leave the room completely for radiation. Her voice came through over the speaker after they'd left me alone.

I breathed through my belly. I could do anything for a few minutes. Soft spa music played over the speakers. I closed my eyes, taking myself to a distant beach. I tried to visualize my special place, in a two-person hammock suspended between palm trees, over-looking the Caribbean, my husband's arms around me. Instead, the machine whirled, and her voice came on to tell me they were starting the radiation. I froze, still for the machine and trying to will myself to relax.

"Beam on," she said.

"Beam me out of here, Scotty," I thought. Take me someplace far away from here.

When the whirring stopped and she told me the radiation beam had ceased, I assumed they were coming to unstrap me.

They didn't.

She'd said something else, but I didn't catch it. I didn't know how to ask her to repeat it with the tongue depressor and mouthpiece in. So I waited, anticipating what might happen next, my muscles tight beneath the hard plastic. The machine moved into a new position, and she told me we shared the Beam with the room next door, and she would be able to turn it back on in 25 seconds.

Okay, 25 seconds isn't long. One more Beam is manageable. But my brain started to ask questions it didn't think of before. How many Beams are there? How long do I stay in the mask? Why hadn't I thought of the right questions to ask?

The 25 seconds ended, and the Beam started. I stayed perfectly still, trying to focus on the imagery of light sabers fighting my tumor, borrowed from a friend who thrived through her own radiation. I gave myself a pep talk, followed by more unanswered questions. How many more Beams were there?

It ended and the machine moved around me again. This time a large square plate lowered to my face. I had been trying to keep my eyes closed but the plate moved slowly towards me, coming at my face. How close would it get? My Anxiety Brain ramped up by the minute. It had questions too. Irrational ones.

The plate stopped above my face, and I knew what she'd say before she said it.

Beam on.

This one pointed right between my eyes. This one fought the tumor head on. I imagined the raindrop in my mind's eye. My breathing slowed. Time slowed. I watched the raindrop, the curve, the mantra. So'Hum. I am.

I exhaled deep into my belly when the machine retracted. But it found another position. How many more?

"I'm just waiting for the Beam. Two minutes until we have the Beam." Two minutes? How many more minutes total? I asked the questions silently and felt along the plastic in my mouth that held my tongue. I tried to back my forehead away from the plastic mesh, but there was nowhere to go on the hardened pad molded to my head shape. I pressed against the metal table. Again, nowhere to go.

The two minutes dragged on. I tried to take myself back to the beach. But the longer I had more questions than answers, the more panicky I felt. My pulse beat in my neck and bounced against the plastic mask.

"Beam on."

I had tucked my tongue back into its desired position and I fixated on freezing for the Beam. I didn't want to swallow. I didn't want to breathe too deeply. I imagined the protons staying concentrated in the right spot.

When the machine moved again, I willed it to move away from me. I willed the table to leave the center of the machine and wheel me out completely. I imagined the fictional Dorothy Gale and the experiments they did on her in one of my favorite childhood movies. She had been strapped in, but the machines malfunctioned and quit. She got away, escaping her torturers. I wanted to get away to Oz. To go see my friends, like Dorothy. It wasn't just the machine. I might not be able to swallow. Santa had brought me a Vitamix for Christmas. He had a sick sense of humor. I tried to swallow but it felt too heavy, like I needed to clear my throat. How long until I could clear my throat?

Her voice came back in an answer to my unasked question. "This is the last one. Beam on."

Beam on. The last one. My throat constricted. I could breathe soon. And swallow. The minutes dragged by and then, "Okay we are coming back in the room."

The male therapist told me he had to mark the mask before he took it off. He took a Sharpie to spots near my ears and mouth, grazing my upper lip and leaving a purple Sharpie freckle among the rest.

Finally, he disconnected the mask from the table, pulling it free. My hand went to my forehead, rubbing the mesh marks in my skin, an imprint of the plastic lattice on my forehead. Bits of my skin had squished through creating a print on my face. A headache had already formed.

I sat up and everything I had been holding in burst free. I cried with relief and dread as I got off the table and told the therapist that I didn't want to come back every day.

I had 34 more treatments.

I took my pity party back to the changing room and continued to cry while I got dressed. Maybe I would feel better just letting it out. Letting it release.

I heard a woman say, "Are you ready to ring the bell?"

More voices gathered in the hallway and then the bell rang out. I threw my shirt on and opened the door. A boy, maybe five or six years old, a blue ball cap over his bald head, stood next to a bell on the wall, surrounded by people in scrubs holding signs that said, "You did it!" "Last day of radiation treatment" and other congratulatory messages.

My tears retreated, sucked back in. My heart ached for a small stranger and for his family going through it with him. He had done it. Someone in scrubs held his radiation mask, a quarter of the size of mine, in a clear, plastic bag with a drawstring. Another crouched in front of him with a big yellow toy truck.

He had done it. I couldn't take my eyes off of his tiny mask. He'd worn it every day, facing his cancer. Maybe he'd been brave. Maybe he'd cried, like me. Maybe we could do both? Standing there watching someone reach the end on my very first day felt symbolic. He had done it.

I could do it, too.

Going to Hell

1991

I was told I was going to hell at age eleven.

Denise held her orange flag by the wooden pole, guiding the backpack-clad children across the street. Together, we were the masters over the corner of Aurora Boulevard and Corona Drive, ferrying our charges across the street safely for thirty minutes after the bell rang. No matter how many children crossed, or how quickly they moved safely past our intersection, we waited out our assigned time. At twelve years old, we were the last ones to leave school, taking off our bright orange belts, and returning the flags until the next day.

Denise and I both took the job seriously. When the flow of kids slackened and eventually dwindled to nothing, we waited for stragglers, checking our watches for the designated return time. Often on days like that, when the job had nearly ended, our most interesting conversations occurred. Denise wasn't in my primary class, but she held the same sacred office, so a level of trust had grown between us right away. We'd both been given the reflective orange belt which put us in the category of "role models" for the sixth grade. This inherent naïve trust is what made me believe her question was reasonable in the first place.

"Have you been saved?" she asked, letting her pole tilt until the orange flag pooled in the sparse Saint Augustine grass and dirt at her feet.

I shrugged. "I don't know. What do you mean, 'saved?'"

Her impatience evident, she rolled her eyes at my question. "If you don't *know*, then you haven't *been* saved. And you know what *that* means?" She put a hand on her hip.

I shook my head. What *did* it mean that I hadn't been saved?

"It means you're going to hell."

Was she even allowed to say that word? A patrol probably shouldn't use the word h-e-l-l.

"I'm not going to hell," I said, echoing her non-role-model word right back at her. "You don't know that." If she could go to heaven and say *hell*, then I could say it too.

She squinted at me. Maybe she couldn't decide if I was an idiot or just pretending to be one. "What I know is that if you aren't saved, you go to hell. And you aren't."

I let my flag drop. I was missing something key, but I didn't know what. *My parents would have had me "saved," wouldn't they? They wouldn't want me to go to hell. Can kids even go to hell?* Hell was reserved for bad people, like robbers and murderers. How could I possibly be going there? I hadn't done anything to qualify for hell. I was a patrol!

Luckily, our duty ended and the time to leave our post and return our flags ended the conversation.

My parents, a Catholic-raised mother and a Southern Baptist-raised father, both departed from their respective churches, which meant I hadn't been raised to believe in hell at all.

At home, I knew the best (only) person to ask was my mother. She would know if I was *really* going to hell. She'd know why I hadn't been "saved."

I had to work up the nerve to ask about h-e-l-l. But the walk home gave me time to think about it and plan my questions. I would be matter-of-fact. I would tell her what happened. She could help me understand.

I walked home with my little brother. He wouldn't know the answer. I might've tried the question on my older brother, but his middle-school hours meant he hadn't come home from school yet. Mom was there when we arrived, her part-time teller job complete for the day.

"Mom, am I going to hell?"

She laughed at the question and didn't even flinch at the word *hell*. "Of course, not. What gave you that idea?"

I shrugged. "A girl at school. She said I was going to hell because I'm not saved."

"Oh, I see." Her laughter stopped. Maybe I had found the right word to let her know the seriousness of the situation. *Saved.* Now I would understand why I hadn't been saved.

"Why wasn't I saved?" I asked. I hoped her answer would explain the meaning for me. Saved from what? That's a question I didn't think to ask.

"Oh, you were." Her serious tone meant she understood.

This surprised me. If I had been saved, wouldn't I have known it? She must have read the confusion on my face.

"Remember when you received Shaktipat from the Guru?" she asked.

Shaktipat. I remembered the intensive I'd attended that summer in the ashram. I remembered the explanation of the Kundalini awakening at the base of my spine. I had imagined it like a golden snake of energy, uncoiling and growing the length of my spine, so it could erupt from the top of my head and tether me to God somehow.

I nodded.

"That's what she meant, when she asked if you'd been saved. You have been."

I felt stupid for not realizing it. I wish I'd known it earlier when that know-it-all Denise told me I was going to hell.

"Some religions call it being 'saved' and other things, but it's the same. It means that you have a blessing that protects you."

I fingered the tulsi beads around my neck. They meant the same. Protection. "Okay. Thanks." And I ran off to play.

The next day, I told Denise, with confidence and indignation, that I *had* been saved and I was *definitely not* going to hell.

I left out the part about the Shaktipat.

Spiritual Kiss
February 2021

Radiation became a routine. Every day, Monday through Friday, at seven a.m. I took off my wool winter coat, shirt and bra, and put on two hospital gowns, one forward, worn as a top during treatment, and one backward, like a boho-open-front-kimono-cardigan in an awful style. Occasionally I used the restroom, but often, I went straight into the women's waiting room and put my things in a locker. The water cooler offered exceptionally cold water, a respite for my dry mouth. I'd fill a paper cup, take a seat, and watch the fireplace loop playing on the television. I would think about my warm blanket. I would sometimes write notes on my phone.

I arrived late that day and sat with my cup of cold water, waiting my turn. A mother in her winter coat, arms laden with belongings, and her tween/young teenage daughter entered the women's waiting room. The mother looked all business; like most mothers at doctor's offices, she had the practical job of getting her daughter changed and carrying all their things. Her daughter moved slower and shook her head. Her shoulders slumped, she made the slow march toward a treatment she didn't want, carrying the telltale signs I'd been working to cover up. The girl wore a black du-rag to cover her bald head and her eyebrows were as sparse as mine. She wore my outfit, matching me in her two hospital gowns. I couldn't tell if she was shaking her head at the chair her mother had selected. Maybe the girl didn't want to sit so close by. Or maybe her head shook in response to something her mother had said before they entered the room. To me, the shaking meant No more. No more treatment. No more of this.

The girl stood in front of her mother, not taking the chair she had been guided to. She looked into her mother's face, her eyes filled with pleading, dread, and fatigue and she did it again, shaking her head gently, the slight movement saying I don't want to go.

I waited to see if her mother would be firm. I watched to see how she might comfort the young girl. I anticipated learning how I might respond if it were my daughter making the march to the radiation table.

Gently, the mother put her forehead on her daughter's. She brought their mystical third eyes together, connected her perception-beyond-ordinary sight to her daughter's, their invisible brow chakras kissing.

Maybe the mother whispered something inaudible. I felt the energy between them, palpable in the waiting room. The mother, loving and steadfast. The daughter, exhausted and scared. Between them, the kind of love that is so pure and so true.

This forehead touch, like the one the monk, robed in burnt orange, had greeted me with at the same age. Maybe her mother's love could transfer through that spiritual kiss, opening the girl to her treatment, giving her what she needed to take the steps into the next room. She was the seer, and the connection passed her sight to her daughter. You are strong. You will heal. You can do this.

They called the girl's name and she left. Maybe I imagined it, but her slow walk looked resolute, as if her mother had transferred courage or resilience in that touch of their foreheads.

I wanted to speak to the mother, but there were no words.

I'm sorry.

I'm sad for you.

This is so hard.

In that moment, I became the mother, leading her daughter in, holding the strong face of resilience and encouragement. I became the daughter, the cancer patient, about to face the metal table again.

If it's possible to hate cancer more than I already do, seeing it in that girl made it so.

They called me next, leading me to face my own metal table. I crumpled my paper cup and tossed it in the bin on my way out. Treatment moved slower than the previous two days. My mouth, dry now from treatments, made it difficult to swallow with the tongue depressor. The mask held tight, and the machine sat quiet. As I waited for the Beam, making an effort to control my breathing, I thought of the girl. I pictured her next door on her metal table, locked in place under her own tight mask and needing the Beam.

There were many days on the table when my meditation brought a mother and her child to me. I practiced at both. Scared, I would see myself as the baby, held in her mother's arms. The warmth protected me. I could be at ease because there were arms around me.

I was not alone. And then I became the mother, holding the child, comforting her. Shh. It will pass.

I could wait. We could all wait. I could stay for an hour or more, my daily headache forming, my jaw clenching the putty mouthpiece in my teeth, if that's what the girl needed. I could be the mother, instead of the cancer patient girl, exuding love and holding still, silenced in place while the Beam does its work in the room next door. I am certain the mother has wished more than once that she could face the Beam in her daughter's place.

Holding Tight
1993

I had planned to wear black tights with my funeral dress. The ill-fitting dress wasn't long enough to cover my unshaved legs. I worried that it wasn't dark enough, blue instead of black, but it was all I had. I had spent the night before the funeral at my best friend's house, getting to know her adult sister and staying by Katie's side through the night. As we were getting dressed, I realized my only pair of tights were marred with a hole and a long run. Not altogether surprising, since I often wore ill-fitting or holed clothing. I usually leaned into it. I could pretend I wasn't poor, just grunge. But I was getting ready for a funeral, and determined to look respectful.

"It doesn't matter," Katie said, "Just wear the dress without the tights."

"But I haven't shaved my legs." Mortified, I couldn't imagine wearing the dress with bare legs. I had only been shaving a year or so by then, and hairy legs were for children and barbarians.

Her cool sister assured me that no one would notice my legs.

I'd told my mom I needed to go to the funeral—for Katie.

I didn't want to go to a funeral, but I wanted to be there for Katie. Even though I knew all her family would come down from Ohio and she would have her brother and dad. She needed me. We had already become the kind of friends who told each other everything, spent every weekend at each other's houses and wrote long notes to each other during classes. Now her mom had died, and my fierce protectiveness and loyalty meant I would go to a funeral by choice, and I would expose my hairy legs to anyone who decided to look.

***

Katie had shown up in my eighth-grade physical science class, brand new to our school. I was determined to befriend her, though I don't remember why. Maybe it had been her Pearl Jam t-shirt or the way she parted her hair. It took a bit to win her over and her skepticism of me just made me try harder. Aware that I came off as odd and goofy, I persisted because I felt something right away—a soul connection that told me we would be friends.

Katie slowly but surely let me in. By the end of September, we were the best of friends. We both supposedly had other "best" friends and the title can certainly be hard-earned at thirteen. So we honored our long-distance BFFs by calling each other by a synonym to "best friends" and in goofy thirteen-year-old style we signed all our notes with "Your Goodest Buddy." Still, we both knew what it meant.

We started spending the weekend at each other's houses. Although I had been reluctant to let people come to our house and see that we were poor, a near-instant trust with Katie allowed me to let her in. At my house, we watched Faces of Death and listened to Adam Sandler's comedy CD. We had freedom, since my mother left for the club every Friday and Saturday night and the run of the house became ours.

At Katie's, we listened to Nirvana and swam in the pool. We stayed in her room or quietly helped ourselves to ice cream and a movie night.

Her mother, weak and ill, never came out of her bedroom. Breast cancer. She'd had a check-up from a suspicion, and everything came back normal. But something wasn't right and by the time she went back to follow up and they found the cancer, it was advanced. Her family , Katie's dad, sick mother, and big brother, had moved to Florida and now her mother stayed in her room, dying.

We hadn't even finished our first semester of eighth grade when her mom died—just over a week before Christmas.

***

My parents had a conversation with us about the divorce before the move happened. Sitting in the living room as they explained how they weren't going to be together anymore, I thought I should maybe fake some sadness about it, since they seemed somber. But all I could think was thank god you won't be fighting and trying to kill each other anymore. When we were invited to ask questions, I only had one. "Can we go outside and play?"

Two months before I met Katie, my mom picked me up from a long bus ride trip home from the Florida Keys. I had been on an overnight field trip with the biology class.

"Do you want to go to a movie?" she asked.

"Sure," I said excitedly. She never offered treats like that. We were too poor for family time at the movies. "Is there something good out?"

"I don't know."

"What do you want to see?" I asked.

"Oh, I can't go. I thought I'd drop you off."

"By myself?"

The alarms started going off. The bizarre conversation meant something else was going on.

She shrugged, gripping the steering wheel and trying to act casual. "I guess we could pick up a friend."

We went back and forth about who to pick up. I wanted to go home and brush my teeth, but she made it clear that we wouldn't go home first, just straight to the movies. I had been on a bus ride for about eight to ten hours. Still, the dangling gift of the movies, a special once-in-a-while treat hung out there and tugged at me. When I asked if we could pick up a neighbor, a girl my age who lived four doors down, she agreed.

"Good, then I can pop in and brush my teeth before we go."

"No. If we go home, we aren't going back out."

The decision felt like a slap. Was I being treated to the movies or not? Furious that I wasn't allowed to go if I wanted to brush my teeth first, I decided I didn't want to go. I refused the movies and told her I just wanted to go home. It had been a long day and the bus ride made me "too gross" to go to the movies with a friend, too insecure to go alone, and too suspicious of what might be happening at home to go at all.

At home, Dad's amp sat in the front room next to stacks of brown boxes and his guitar cases. Coming home to the moving boxes meant Dad had cleared out his belongings and much of the meditation room. His guitars and books were packed.

I didn't understand why Mom might think the movies were a better alternative. Maybe she wanted to keep the memory of stacked boxes, the transitional moment of their break, away from me. I don't remember where my brothers were—maybe over at a friend's house. Whether we were there to see it or not—Dad was leaving. And her coup to hide it from me only made me suspicious of her. She couldn't tell me the truth, so she tried to fabricate a gift for me, one that was nearly irresistible.

***

Grief carves holes in memories. My memory of that time is like a porous piece of coral. The whole is there, but the missing spaces feel as important as the concrete and tangible. It wasn't as if we sank into a black hole, an abyss of grief. Maybe because we were tethered so tightly together, I thought; and I held us above the water. In ordinary ways, life after Katie's mom died looked the same as life before she died. We walked to the Food Lion and bought our obsession, a brand-new ice cream flavor called Chocolate Chip Cookie Dough. Then, into Video Depot where we rented our weekend movies. We snuck Basic brand cigarettes from her dad's secret stash and shared them in the backyard as part of our angry rebellion against the world. We swam in the pool on warm days for hours, listening to a constant stream of Soundgarden, Smashing Pumpkins and Weezer. Some days that music was too happy and we turned to Nine Inch Nails and Rage Against the Machine to feed our anger instead.

Anger came easier than sadness and helped us cope. Anger satiated more easily. Still, there were nights that I crawled out of the rollaway bed and into Katie's narrow twin bed when a nightmare came, and her sobbing couldn't be soothed.

It wasn't until Marcos held me in my own grief around my cancer diagnosis that I realized how grief has formed me. For years I didn't understand why I didn't enjoy sad movies or why I thought it was appropriate and necessary to hide my tears. For all of my adulthood, I've harbored a secret fear that if I opened the door to sadness, it would flood out and consume me and I would never be able to recover. So I spent a lot of time holding that door closed.

I met cancer again in the years since I watched it take my best friend's mom. It took two of my grandparents during my teens, and I wasn't the least bit surprised. That's what cancer did. The idea that someone could recover from their cancer seemed completely alien.

Before we understood that this cancer, my cancer, could be cured, it felt like a death sentence.

Rare.

Aggressive.

Stage Four.

There were nights that uncontrolled sobbing spilled from me and there was nothing Marcos could do but hold me. I was Cai, at the ashram to heal my cancer, or maybe to die in peace. I was my grandmother, lying weak in bed, taking the tulsi beads from my son, listening to him play guitar as I died. I was thirteen again and cancer meant that I would stay in my room, and it would spread. It wouldn't heal and my children would be motherless like Katie. I prayed that someone would be there for them.

***

One night at Katie's, we stood in the dark, outside the screened pool with a single cigarette between us, passing it back and forth as if it were a joint. Every time we puffed, we got light-headed, the red light a beacon calling us. On this evening, or maybe another just like it, I broke into a complete tirade. Self-indulgent anger had long since become my identity, evident in my combat boots and rebellious attitude.

I don't remember exactly what my rant had been on that particular night. Probably that I hated my parents. They had ruined my life. My mother had become more and more unbearable since my father left. He had disappeared into his new life and girlfriend. His presence became less, and then so did hers. I was somehow even more broken by their dissolved relationship. I had taken their broken marriage into my identity. Now I amounted to more than the girl with ill-fitting clothes or the teen on free lunches. I became all of that, plus the kid with divorced parents who couldn't cut it in honors classes anymore. My mother had decided that she'd do everything she should have done before marrying my father at eighteen and I despised her for it.

Katie took the tirade in stride. She let me vent and listened for a while. But I crescendoed into a whine that was finally too much.

She flicked the cigarette when she'd had enough. "Well at least you still get to go see your dad on weekends. My mom died. She's gone. So as bad as it is, it's not that bad."

Her words stunned me, and I quieted. At least I had a mom to hate and a dad to resent. I supposed I should be glad for that. No matter how awful, they were alive. But were they? Katie had a hole where her mother used to be. And I spent what was left of my childhood filling it as often as I could.

Her mother disappeared into cancer. My mother disappeared into her own grief and loss. Her mother became ashes. Mine became eighteen again.

In the end, it wasn't me holding Katie up in her grief after all, but our mutual need for someone to mother us. So we both held on tight, our grip on each other the only real thing we had left.

Dinnertime

Radiation 2021

Amy's Soups
Nettle Tea
Popsicles, eight different brands
Applesauce
Hummus
Almond butter
Smoothie ingredients
Fruit, all kinds
Vegan macaroni and cheese
Coconut water
Protein powder
V8 Drinks
Yogurt
Ripple protein shakes
Sweet Earth cauliflower mac and cheese

The grocery bill was fairly high for two people, considering that many of the options went uneaten.

"Do you think you might like some artichoke hearts? You love those." Marcos had the laptop poised on his lap, trying to make a grocery delivery order.

"Eww," I groaned.

"I know you like macaroni as a comfort food. Will you try it?"

"I couldn't swallow it last time."

He ordered it anyway. Of the popsicles, only one flavor of one brand became the option I could stomach. It took eight variety boxes to find it.

I'd lost thirty pounds on purpose before the diagnosis. I had arrived at a healthy, post-kids mom body and a weight I was happy to maintain. But as the cancer treatment pressed on, the scale ticked down more and more. I had never been so unhappy to lose weight. I knew I looked ill. Bald, skinny, pale, the radiation burns standing out on my face and neck against my pale, freckled skin.

"You've got to eat more. How much did you weigh this week?"

"I'm down twenty pounds since cancer."

"So, fifty total?" he asked.

I nodded weakly.

We saw the nurse practitioner that week, short and spunky and always in laced-up boots. Practical for winter, her look gave her the appearance of someone who would kick your ass. I came to think of her as my "cancer midwife," though, because she had a gentle spirit. She recognized my anxiety over trying new things and every time she suggested a countermeasure for cancer side effects, she guided me into it with a full explanation and even walked and talked me through the specifics of several comforts and cures.

But that day, when she saw my weight and talked to us about my diet, she met Marcos' eyes with a meaningful stare.

"It's okay for now, but we don't want to see these drastic dips in weight. And your body still needs nutrition outside of your hydration days."

The two of them had a discussion about feeding tubes while I closed my eyes and took deep breaths, willing the conversation away. That afternoon, back in the little apartment on 63rd, he begged me to eat. "I need you to think about what you can do to eat. I need you to be so hungry that you can power through. Do you think you could try more of the medical marijuana? I don't think you've been even close to a therapeutic dose yet."

"But then I'm going to get high," I argued.

"I don't care if I have to call you Snoop Dog for the next two months; I need you to eat. Trust me, I did the research. You do not want a feeding tube. And if you keep losing weight, we are going to lose the privilege of avoiding it."

I had listened to my oncologist and obtained a prescription for medical marijuana. Marcos had walked me through the steps, set up appointments, and filled out all the paperwork with me. Once it had been approved, he drove me down to the dispensary. I went in alone, as I had for much of the cancer treatment itself.

I spent an hour talking to the pharmacist about what a square I am and about how I don't want to feel like my head has floated away. We talked about how sensitive I am to medications and what I needed to accomplish if the time came—appetite, sleep, anxiety—

all in anticipation of what the cancer treatment might do to me. I did not mention the plants that had grown in my parents' closet, the smell of the master bathroom, or the desire I had to never become them.

Through the induction chemotherapy, I allowed myself CBD. When that didn't work, I began a THC tincture under the tongue. Afraid of it, I let Marcos give me a single drop the first time. Later when I threw up from the chemotherapy load, I blamed the tincture. In the dispensary, we talked through my hesitation, the option of edibles and how to control the dosing. She convinced me that vaporizing it would allow for the most control over the dose. It wasn't going to combust, so it wouldn't have the same effect as "smoking," but it works quickly and would allow for me to find the "lowest therapeutically effective dose" for my body. It would also allow me to add more when needed without it being a train I couldn't get off, as I feared the edibles would be.

Marcos handed me an army green device that looked like an open-top canteen. "Here's your smoke buddy." You just blow into that to absorb the smell and all. I wondered what my parents' bathroom would have smelled like if they'd had one. "Remember, if you hate it, you've just got to sleep. But please try."

I took the first drag on the vape pen, watching the end light up. I had tried it a couple of times by now, but only one or two puffs. This time, I decided to keep going. Three. Four. Five. Six.

This time I let it come. My throat had an open sore that burned like fire when I swallowed. I began creating spittoons with paper cups to avoid swallowing my own saliva. I couldn't bear that he might have to wash a cup full of my saliva, so I'd asked for paper.

He made nettle tea, a recommendation from my acupuncturist. The warm liquid soothed my throat. He brought me an ice water. Very hot or extremely cold were the only ways for me to swallow. The TV lit up, Gordon Ramsay encouraged the participants to fight for their spot on MasterChef, weeding them out one by one. But my favorite part was watching them cook, hearing them describe it, and seeing Graham Elliot close his eyes when he took a bite of food, shutting out the world to experience only what he had in his mouth. I didn't expect to enjoy food the way he did or the way I'd enjoyed it before. I just wanted to be able to swallow it.

My eyelids were heavy. I opened my phone and started to scroll for food. There had to be something I wanted to eat. I thought something soft and warm might be best for my throat. So I told Marcos I needed some "Italian grandmama bread." When he asked what I meant by "Italian grandmama bread" I described for him a handmade loaf, fresh from the oven, warm, made with the expertise of wrinkly hands and everlasting love. "You know, Italian grandmama bread," I said again, as if the shorthand meant the same for him. It wasn't as if I had my own Italian grandmama back home, but we were in New York City, and I had to imagine I would find some authentic bread somewhere.

I began the hunt for a bakery and came up short. We were far north of Little Italy, and I couldn't find a close bakery. Magnolia Bakery popped up for me and is supposed to have the best banana pudding in the city. I ordered some. Not sure how I'd feel about all the bananas and cream, I added a chocolate pudding to be on the safe side. Plus they had cookies. I wanted those too.

I went back to looking for Italian bread, but nothing else at an Italian restaurant would sit right. Too acidic. Too tough, too heavy. I ended up placing a grocery order. A loaf of Italian bread from the grocery store bakery. A frozen loaf of garlic bread. A French baguette in case the Italian bread wasn't soft enough. An order of dinner rolls if all else failed.

I had become hungry waiting for the food to arrive. The door to the street remained locked at all times, so the phone rang every time someone came with a delivery. Magnolia Bakery. Grocery store #1, Grocery Store #2, and an order of soup from the vegan place on the corner.

Marcos had fallen asleep and the third ringing for delivery woke him. He pulled the groceries in and unpacked. "What did you order?"

"I don't know. I wasn't sure what I would be able to eat."

"Which one do you want to start with?"

The sound of warm garlic bread sounded best and he suggested putting in half the loaf.

"No. Put in the whole loaf."

"You don't need the whole loaf. There's no way you are going to eat that."

But on my insistence, he put the whole loaf in. Grocery store frozen garlic bread requires both sides of the loaf to create the perfect, soft, moist center, and there was no way to separate the frozen halves without compromising the center. So he baked the whole loaf. I wished I could smell the bread baking, but my smell had gone and would not likely ever return.

The foot-long bread loaf came out, crusty on the outside, soft and warm on the inside. I had my ice water, my hot tea, my mouthwash, my appetite stimulant, and Master Chef started on the TV.

Slowly I scraped the soft middle from the outer edges, creating an empty crusty boat. I took small bites, eating slowly, careful with my throat. When I had scraped clean one side of the bread, Marcos took the rest, enjoying for himself "the best part" and offered me the other half. I said yes and took it, repeating the process, until only an empty crust of bread remained.

We were both shocked at how much I ate.

"That's more than you've eaten all week." he said.

I reached over and squeezed his hand. "Thanks for making me get high."

He squeezed it back, "No problem, Snoop."

Vanity

April 2021

In middle school, Katie "helped" me with my eyebrows. Luckily, they weren't as overplucked as most of the 90s brows, simply because of the way they grew. I had no idea how to use a brow pencil to fill them in and they didn't have the look of the "popular girl brows" because they simply wouldn't.

Vanity is a luxury for beautiful people. Growing up, the beautiful people were the popular girls. I leaned into the "alt rock/prog rock/ dirt rocker" grunge look of the 90s. If the grunge bands I loved so deeply could look good in t-shirts, ripped jeans, and shit-kickers, so could I. It was good camouflage: *I'm not poor,* it said; *I just don't give a fuck.* That attitude got me through middle and high school.

At my first "real" job, I had to dress business casual. Being nearly six feet tall and fashion-ignorant meant I had to find clothes that fit and didn't come out of my grunge wardrobe. It was the late 90s and early 2000s, and I promptly made my way to the men's section of a department store and bought pleated dockers and golf shirts. It became my work uniform. I didn't know how to dress "like a girl" and I just needed to avoid the daily purgatory of choosing an outfit.

In my mind, I had met the requirements to dress for work, and that had to be good enough. A friend and coworker asked me once if she could dress me and help me with my outfits. *You can't wear baggy on top of baggy. Are these men's pants? An empire waist looks amazing on you. What would you think about a blouse instead of...that? You're so tall, you'd look fabulous in a dress once in a while. Do you have any options besides these men's shoes?* While I appreciated the sentiment and guidance during our one and only shopping trip, I still had no idea how to dress myself or the budget to do so.

Before I knew it, I needed maternity clothes. For the first time, I allotted a small part of my paycheck to fashion and dressed more feminine out of necessity. Men's clothes did not have adequate room for my pregnant body. The waists of my slacks had grown too tight. The long men's dockers didn't come in maternity, after all. Once the baby arrived, I leaned heavily into the new-mom look—jeans, a t-shirt, and often at least one article splattered with spit-up.

In my mid-30s, I discovered the eyebrow pencil. With the advent of social media, perception shifted from in-person to pictures and I hated the way my eyebrows looked like they didn't grow all the way to the edge of my brow bone. So I started filling in the latter half of the brow to make the arc complete. I worked to ensure they looked natural since I didn't wear any other daily makeup. I had gone for department store makeovers before, but mostly because they were free, not because I had any intention of buying anything from the heavily perfumed counters. Makeup came from drug stores and were reserved for date nights only. For years, I filled in my brows in the morning, simply because I preferred the way my face looked with complete brows.

After nearly fifteen years of the mom-look, I finally decided to invest in myself and my wardrobe. I joined a style-for-you company that sent me outfits curated by a stylist each month. I started understanding color schemes and mixing and matching outfits. I still turn to jeans and a blouse (sometimes even a t-shirt) often, but the grunge wardrobe and nursing bras are gone, and I own boots in more than one style and scarves for days. I learned how to layer and accessorize just a bit too. At nearly forty, I had finally evolved a personal style that amounted to more than camouflage or practicality.

Then, I became a cancer patient.

I liked my hair. I wanted my brows to look good. I wanted makeup. I didn't want to see myself sick, browless, hairless. The week after my diagnosis I called a brow person to see if I could go for microblading. But the timing of chemotherapy meant that applying the permanent pigment might be too much for my immune system.

I told my kids, "When I look like shit and feel like shit, I need you to straighten my wig and put on my eyebrows." They laughed. But I meant it. Maybe if I felt shitty enough, I wouldn't care about my eyebrows, but I didn't want to imagine feeling that bad.

We went wig shopping before my hair started to fall out. I've barely worn the wigs, but I love them anyway. I want to look normal and feel normal and when people see me without hair, they *know*. Some days I want to tell the whole world: I am fighting. This is how I fight. But other days, I want to blend in and just look like a middle-aged woman with worries about her kids, and job, and appointments.

I made it almost all the way through cancer treatment without publicly sharing a picture of myself looking like a cancer patient.

I shared a picture of my shaved head in defiance, but it had been carefully curated. I had on makeup and earrings and still a bit of short, cute hair remaining on my head.

Then treatment started. At first, I only shared pictures of myself with my wigs on. Slowly, it became clear that I wasn't going to wear those to doctors' appointments and chemotherapy, and the beanies became my go-to head gear. But with my glasses and eyebrows on, I still didn't look sick. During chemo weeks when I looked a little rough, I shared pictures of our dogs instead.

When I felt well, I filled my eyebrows in. As the weeks wore on, I had to fill them in more and more until finally radiation started and obliterated them completely.

Everyone has seen a cancer patient, if not in person, at least on TV. The bald head. The missing eyebrows. The tired eyes. It's not difficult to pinpoint if you see someone with those features. Before long, there they were, staring back at me from my mirror.

I got too sick to put my eyebrows on every day. And then my skin burnt so badly during radiation that I couldn't have put them on if I'd wanted to. A red flare between my eyes, the sides of my neck peeling where they'd targeted the lymph nodes.

So I walked around New York City eyebrowless and didn't care about the gaze of a stranger passing me in the street. But I still never shared a photo where friends and family could see it.

Marcos's cousin, an oncologist at MSK, was the first person I knew to see me without eyebrows. He and his wife came to bring us dinner, offering love, support, and food during treatment. Absurdly, I said to my husband, "but I don't have eyebrows," and Marcos reassured me they wouldn't mind.

I still didn't post pictures.

I went to my doctor's appointments without eyebrows during the worst part of the burns. Once I got too hot and had to pull my beanie off. I sat there with Marcos and the nurse practitioner, and it was okay in there because she'd seen it all before.

The radiation burns peeled, and my skin felt brand new, if also raw. Some of the more difficult side effects of radiation began to heal and I started feeling well enough to put my eyebrows on. I had made it through the worst part, I thought.

Dizzy and sick after my final round of chemotherapy, my temperature climbed, I vomited, my blood pressure dropped, and I fainted. It was day four of my hospitalization before my husband could finally visit me. As soon as he had his shoes off, he was in the hospital bed with me, holding me. And when he pulled out his phone with a look of joy on his face, I let him take the picture. It wasn't the first picture I'd taken without eyebrows. I'd documented my radiation burns in a daily private photo shoot. But letting someone else take my picture meant letting him share if he wanted to. And he did.

When I saw the image of myself in a social media feed, smiling at my husband, I wanted my first thought to be about how happy I was to see him. But my gaze immediately went to my eyebrows, and I cringed at the idea of everyone seeing me like that.

It's more than me being sick or looking like a cancer patient. It's more than me turning into the kind of woman who doesn't want to be seen without makeup. As much as it pains me to admit it, I have bought into the idea that women are supposed to look a certain way: feminine, attractive, desirable. Even writing it makes me cringe—and worse, question who I thought I was. I raised my kids to be feminists. I'm not shallow. I've taught them that "it's what's on the inside that counts." I have even said, "you aren't your body" like my mother used to say to me. But sitting here bald and eyebrowless, it's hard to believe those words.

Bald is beautiful. I haven't judged others for being bald, so why am I so harsh on myself? And if eyebrows make me feel normal, then I can draw them on. But does it really change the world if someone sees me without them? Why would I care less about someone seeing me go out braless than eyebrowless?

My obsession with my eyebrows isn't about eyebrows or vanity. It's about not seeing myself look sick and not letting others see me that way either.

I am strong. I am a fighter. I am smart. I am a good mother. I am funny. I am a good wife. I am kind. I am a good friend. I am creative. I am a hard worker. I am loving.

It's true: I am not this body. Or maybe I am more than this body. I live inside it for now, but this collection of skin, muscle, sinew, organs, and bones is not who I am. This tumor is not who I am.

Sharing Clothes

1995

We had reduced-fee lunches, one running vehicle (only because of my grandmother's generosity), and a run-down, roach-infested house my parents had somehow managed to buy when I was eight. Dad had packed up his guitar and left two years before, taking with him the restraint that had held my mother back. For the first time in her life, she had a full-time job and had started hanging out with a twenty-something crew. I entered high school and my mother turned forty. As luck would have it, we wore the same size. Asking a fifteen-year-old to share a wardrobe with her mother felt embarrassing enough, but our lack of funds meant I shared her clothes or went without. Sure, I had a few birthday-gifted t-shirts of the Nirvana and Pearl Jam variety that she didn't touch, but the rest was fair game. Besides that, nothing belonged to me, and I wore whatever we shared.

On an October day, she had planned one of her regular nighttime outings on a school night. Maybe it had been Mondays for Old Wave Night at the Milk Bar. It could have been Ladies night at some local night club or a concert. At fifteen, I justified her choices to myself. It must've been hard for her to marry at eighteen, to move straight from her father's home to her husband's. She had lived in the country surrounded by rednecks. It had been her only way out. I used to think she wasn't that smart—but maybe it was just the opposite. I justified who she became when my dad pulled out of the driveway for good and she went off the deep end. She never had a chance to do all those things she should've done at eighteen. She had to do them now despite her newly broken family and children at home. I told myself that while I cooked boxed macaroni and powdered cheese on the third night that week for my little brother. I told myself that when I locked the door behind her at ten o'clock and watched MTV until I went to bed, many hours before she arrived back home. I told myself that when I woke up in the morning and put on the dirty jeans that she had promised to wash and leave over the dining room chair for me to wear to school.

In my house, being fifteen meant I could take care of myself. I could eat my cold Cheerios, pack my school bag, and see myself out the door while she slept. Katie picked me up in her hand-me-down white hatchback. I loved that I never had to take the school bus or rely on my mother. Every day, without fail, Katie showed up in my driveway and delivered me away from that house and that life to a place where I could be *me*.

That day started the same as every morning. We went straight to the band room to meet up with the rest of our friends. Anyone who had brought their instrument home for practice could return it to a shelf to store until band class. My piccolo stayed in my backpack, but storage was a must-have for those who played the sousaphone, tenor sax, or trombone.

I went straight to the tuba room to kiss my boyfriend, Noah, a tall tuba player with the smile of a game show host. In our kissing hideaway, among the smell of brass instrument oil and leather cases, I discovered a lump in the pocket of the jeans my mother had worn to the club the night before. She'd taken them off in the early hours of the morning and placed them over the chair while the rest of the house slept. She'd been in no condition to get up in the morning, much less wash them or remember to check the pockets.

How had I missed it before? In my early morning, Cheerios-eating, quick-dressing routine, I had slipped on the jeans in a rush, grabbed my backpack and headed out the door.

I pulled the wadded bulge out. In my hand, I held a baggie with a lump of greens.

Marijuana.

I had never seen it in real life before—only in one of those scare-tactic, anti-drug films in health class. Or maybe I had seen it in a movie or heard of it in a song. And there it sat, in my very own hand.

My stomach dropped. I looked up into my boyfriend's wide eyes. He'd seen it too. He stood with his back to the window in the door to the five-by-eight tuba room and looked at me, confused. "What are you doing with that?"

"Holy shit. Holy shit." The frozen moment of bewilderment jolted into reality that I stood on school grounds with a fistful of drugs. "This isn't mine. My mom—she borrowed my jeans." I couldn't decide if it embarrassed me more to share clothes with her (and wear them used, dirty) or that I was in deep shit, holding a wad of drugs in my palm.

Noah took the baggie out of my hands. I didn't know what constituted a lot or little of it. I had no idea how marijuana was measured or sold. But the wad was nearly as thick as a Taco Bell bean burrito. *How had I missed it?* He shoved it into his tuba locker and sealed it in. "Your mom is a real piece of shit, you know."

I looked down. "I know."

"I'm going to hold onto this until after school. You could get expelled."

"You could get expelled!" I knew my protest was too little, too late. Noah was a senior. I was a sophomore. I'd been in high school just a little over two months, after spending my freshman year at the junior high. I'd never had more than a middle-school romance. Is that what boyfriends were supposed to do? Were they supposed to protect you by taking your mom's drugs and stashing them in their locker, putting themselves on the line?

We argued for each other's well-being for a few minutes. In the end, he took me by my shoulders and looked down at me with his piercing blue eyes. "I can handle this. I'm about to graduate and get out of here. You have your whole high school in front of you. You can't let something like this fuck things up for you. It'll be fine. I'll hold it and I'll come home with you after school. We'll deal with it then."

He was planning a confrontation. I secretly looked forward to my boyfriend berating my mother. I wanted to imagine someone standing up for me. That ended the conversation. He kissed me again. He had a pouty lower lip that he always sucked in before he kissed me. It made for kind of a sloppy kiss, but I didn't care. I just knew that it was the perfect way to kiss.

"I'll see you after first period."

With that, I left for Geometry. I hated first period. By the end of sophomore year, it had become the only class I'd ever failed. But in October, I had still been struggling through it. If I'd known then that I would have to sit through it again in summer school, I might have worried less at the time.

But that day Geometry was the last thing on my mind. And when Mrs. Hollis called on me, I didn't have the faintest idea what the answer might be. I couldn't summon the proper mortification either because the burrito of drugs in my boyfriend's locker was an axe that could come down on our heads at any moment. *What was the likelihood that the school would have random locker checks today? What was the likelihood that it would be one of the infamous dog-sniffing days? Would the drugs be safer in the band room or out in the main hall of lockers? If there were locker checks, would that include the band room lockers? What if they found the drugs? Would Noah be expelled? Would I? Would my mother be reported to DCF? Would they take us away from her and move us in with our dad? He and his new wife had a house, but they lived all the way across town, and I would have to change schools.* As much as I would've loved to see my mother punished for her poor life choices, I didn't want to pay the price with my own future.

Geometry ended and I made my way back to the band room. I didn't find Noah in any of the usual places—outside by the picnic tables, in the breezeway that led toward the gym, or the concert room.

Through the closed door to the tuba room, I could hear muffled voices. I opened the door and slipped in, closing it behind me to stop the noise from carrying, but my presence didn't stop the argument.

"She's *my* mother and *my* sister, so it's *my* problem. I don't need your help." My brother shouted at Noah. My brother amounted to only a hundred and forty-five pounds soaking wet, but he had spirit. However, the fact that he looked like Opie from the Andy Griffith show made his brave stand somewhat comical.

"And she's *my* girlfriend. And it's *my* problem when we are standing at *my* locker and she pulls a wad of weed out of her pocket. She could be expelled. Your piece-of-shit mother is going to hear it from me today. What the fuck is her problem?"

"What the fuck is *your* problem? This is not your fight, Noah. No one needs you to put on a cape and save the day. So just hand the shit over and we'll be done here." His speech was slightly weakened by the fact that he had to look up into Noah's face, who was a head taller, to give it.

"I already took care of it. So let's just leave it alone until after school."

"You guys..." My voice drowned in the next shout. My presence might have been fueling the testosterone-driven pissing match. I couldn't fight them myself, like the time I had tried propelling my way back to shore, caught in the current. I never found the sandy bottom. My brother had yanked me back to the surface.

My brother lowered his voice and stepped back. He held out his hand. "I'm not going to say it again. It's not your fight. Hand it over and I will deal with it. And you can say whatever you want to my mom after school. Please." *Please.* My brother was a junior, so the high school hierarchy placed him below Noah. Maybe he needed the *please* to get through.

Noah looked back and forth between us. I gave a half-shrug, half-nod. He opened his locker and pulled it out, shoving it into my brother's chest. "This better never happen again. Next time, I go to the principal myself." He poked my brother in the chest with a long slender finger.

"Okay. Thank you." My brother left the tuba room triumphant as he left to put the drugs away (again).

Noah's flushed cheeks puffed out as he exhaled heavily and shook his shaggy, golden hair. I collapsed into his chest, fighting back tears. Tears of anger. Tears of shame. Tears of relief at being held and comforted by the only person who felt normal in my life. I didn't win the fight and the tears came. He held me, rubbing my back and telling me it would be okay.

Our seven short minutes ended and I had to get to American History. I didn't care about the revolution or the war or whatever Mrs. Spencer went on about. I just wanted the clock to wind faster, like in a movie, and flash straight to after school. But I didn't want to go home. My stomach filled with acid and dread. My brother had come through when I thought I might not make it back to shore. He'd yanked me out of the current when I had been too tired to swim. He'd always been my lifeguard.

Ten minutes into the lecture and note-taking routine, there was a knock on the classroom door. Mrs. Spencer paused mid-sentence, pushed the door open and took a note from the hands of a student aid. "Sita, can you come here, please?"

My stomach flipped. A wave of nausea flowed over me.

Oh God. They've found the drugs. My brother's told them everything. The principal wants me. The police are here. DCF is here. I will have to move and change schools because my mother is unfit. The department of children and families don't take kindly to burrito-sized drug packages in a teenager's pocket, especially if they belong to her mother.

I swallowed hard and stood. I imagined in that moment collapsing onto the floor, but my feet somehow stayed beneath me. I would not get out of it that easily. I made my way to the door, weak and faint-hearted.

Mrs. Spencer pushed the door open and held it for me. I stepped in the hall expecting the school officer to be there, waiting to escort me to a holding cell or something. And there, in the hallway, stood my mother. She waited until Mrs. Spencer went back into the classroom and the student aid rounded the corner at the end of the hall. Without so much as a greeting or a single word to me, she lunged forward, hands diving into each of my pockets, searching.

I held up my empty hands, palms facing her as she frisked me. My fear flashed to anger and I stepped back. "I don't have your shit." I emphasized the word *shit*. It was the first time I had ever sworn in front of her.

"Where is it?" Her dark, wild eyes flashed like a caged animal's.

"That's what you care about? Not, 'Gee, I sure hope I didn't endanger you at school or anything. Gee, I'm so sorry I was too drugged out to remember to hide my stash before you took your jeans back. Or how about, sorry I didn't wash your jeans like I promised.' Nothing like that? I could be *expelled* for this."

She stared me down. "I'm sorry," she said woodenly. "Where is it?"

Her concern and focus were elsewhere. I explained how it had gone from my pocket to my boyfriend's locker, and on to my brother that morning.

She looked around frantically. Her eyes were sunken and bulging at the same time. She looked up the hall, then down again. "Where is he?" She had nothing to say about Noah, the locker, or the exchange of drugs between three students (including two of her own children) in the first two hours of school. Just *where is he* so she could find her stash.

If there had ever been a chance to mock her without getting slapped, that was the moment. I smiled condescendingly at her. It gave me a sick pleasure to see her struggle. "I have no idea. I don't know what he has second period. I guess that means you have to go back to the front office and tell them you pulled your wrong kid out of class. And then what? You'll walk him to the band room, interrupt *another* class and open his locker to get your stuff? Smart. I have a class to be in. Try not to get caught."

I turned my back on her and went back into the classroom. By the time I reached my seat, and turned back toward the door, the rectangular window was empty. She had gone back down the hall. Back to the office. I didn't know how she might explain that one to the office staff.

I'd like to say that I gained some kind of grace or favor with my mother after her mishap. But that's not what happened. I'd like to say I took off those jeans after school and burned them in defiance. But that's not what happened either. I couldn't afford to ruin a good pair of jeans when I only had two.

That summer I started my first job within a week of turning sixteen. And I never had to share clothes with her again.

Closed

May 2021

I go to the ashram's website first—everything is scheduled, booked
and planned through the internet these days. Unlike others,
I hadn't been handed a gift at the airport. I didn't hear about it
through a long-haired friend as my parents had. Instead, I had
grown up in the presence of the Guru.

She was everywhere and nowhere. The image of her lived on our
altar. We met regularly with other devotees to listen to her talks,
to chant, to meditate and eat together. We went to their homes.
I was always fascinated to see the inside of other peoples' homes.
Which room did they use for their temple? What did their altar
look like? But more importantly, did they have children I could play
with? Was there anyone else in their home who was also there
by adjacency?

I wasn't sure what I believed, but I was a joiner. So I chanted with
my heart. I took meditation seriously. I thanked the host for having us.

The blurry image of my parents sharpened over the years. And the
more I saw the truth of them, the blurrier their beliefs became.

I floated away from the ashram where I'd spent a whole summer living. The altar had been taken down after dad moved out. The visits with other devotees became less frequent. Dad became a Buddhist. Mom became a hard and unforgiving person.

But the remnants of the words I had chanted stayed with me. I could recall the mantras as easily as memorized nursery rhymes. And when I faced my life-or-death moment, I returned to the teachings of the Guru.

Their website is a modern-day brochure. I can learn about the Guru there. I can purchase things from their bookstore. I can navigate to the page about the ashram where I lived. I can see an image of the forest rimming the lake where I used to explore and play.

When I try to plan a visit, I am taken in a circle, where I can learn more about the practices. Finally, I click the link to offer seva. A gift of full-time practice to offer selfless service to the Guru—that appears to be the only way in.

I call.

No one answers. I leave a message.

When my call is finally returned, I explain myself. "I grew up with the practices of the Guru. I have lived at the ashram. I just want to visit—walk the grounds."

"How long has it been since you practiced?"

I explain my cancer, my way back into meditation. I explain that I only want to take a walk, see the lake, move through the forest where I climbed and played and hid. If possible, I'd love to walk through the hall where I meditated and slept in my mother's lap, see the dorm where we lived.

She is curt. She does not meet my cancer news the way most people do. Her tone does not change. There is no empathy.

"Can you offer seva to the Guru?"

"Well I am not asking to come live there. I have a family. I just want to visit."

"The Ashram is not open to visitors." She says the word visitors as if it were "intruders." I have become an Outsider. Maybe that is what I want to be, after all. How could the ashram be closed to me?

I imagine driving to their gates. I can see the exterior of their compound, closed and locked—the property behind the gate an oasis that is not for me. I imagine myself standing outside the gate—feeling my otherness. I am reminded of the book of quotes from the Guru. "Remember: wherever you are, God is. We all live in God's heart."

I drive to a trail, I take my own path into the woods, my meditation shawl in hand. I do not need the ashram to meditate. I do not need the ashram to validate.

Life in the Water

June 2021

"It's really over," they said. The fervor in their voices froze me. I nodded and confirmed it. "It's over."

I meant the treatment. They meant the cancer.

But will it ever be over?

I want normal. Don't you want to hear about the weather and my family or something that isn't about staring death in the face?

But normal is an illusion.

The next scheduled scan is like a dark storm cloud rolling in. The days tick by. Whatever is happening in my head, with my cancer, will be revealed. That doesn't mean it isn't happening now. That doesn't mean that the next scan will be the decider. But, for me, there will always be a before and an after.

The before: I trusted my body. I was young, still raising my family, loving my husband, driving to pick up groceries, surviving a pandemic, grading papers.

The after: I will never *not* be a cancer patient now. It's like motherhood. There is the before and the after (really the *during*).

The moment I became pregnant, I entered a club of other women. Then when I gave birth and held the wet newborn against my skin, I experienced something that marked me. It moved me from maiden to mother. I looked at that baby and my mind was blown. Love had been a word. A word I thought I had understood that took on a new meaning. One look at the baby and I understood what love meant for the first time in my life. I realized I had never loved anyone. Not my parents, not my siblings, not my friends, and not the man who made that baby with me.

You can never go home again. Too much has changed. It will never be the place that it was because time passes, and things change. I can never be the maiden again. I know too much. I moved into motherhood, and it marked me. I'm etched with everything that happened to me in the nearly-twenty years that followed. Motherhood is the smell of my milk, the silky soft skin of my children, the blood and tears I wiped, dirty fingers I cleaned, driving to school, listening to a heart breaking. There aren't enough words to explain everything that makes up mothering.

And now I live in the *after* of my diagnosis. But it's the *during my life as a cancer patient* that will never end. Like motherhood. One day I get coffee, read a good book, interview for a job, correct myself on the wrong pronoun for my teen, drive my son to the museum, encourage art therapy and hug a friend. Then the next day, I can't move from the couch. My jaw aches, the pain shoots into my neck, my feet are made of pins and needles, my hands are cold and then suddenly, I'm throwing the blanket off, wiping the sweat that has formed beneath my breasts and asking why.

I go to therapy, and we talk about the islands. I swim from island to island. I tell a friend about this lovely and terrible place of the islands. The in-betweens in the water, struggling to get to the next momentary place of safety. And she says, "Life is lived in the water." That explains why I feel like I'm drowning.

Marcos says he feels hopeful about the scans. But he doesn't want to take down the Welcome Home/Fuck Cancer banner that decorates our house. He says we should have the Fuck Cancer party after the scan instead of before. He pretends he wants to pinch pennies this month, but maybe he's holding his breath too. He must see the clouds. I know he wants the all-clear first. But how will we celebrate ever again if there's any gray on the MRI or any illumination on the PET scan?

We hadn't braced for the news before. And somehow bracing feels important now. So I am coiled. Tight, like a sea snake, waiting in a defensive position to strike if I must.

.

Colophon

The cover of *Vanishing Shoals* was set in Roslindale Variable Italic and Ruzicka Freehand. Designed by David Jonathan Ross, Roslindale is a serif typeface that follows in the footsteps of De Vinne, originally published in the 1890s by the Central Type Foundry and named for the famed nineteenth century printer. It's an oldstyle that can't shake its Victorian sensibilities, with sharp, stubby serifs, bulbous terminals, and the occasional hint of diagonal stress. Derived from 1935 sketches by Rudolph Ruzicka, which were discovered in 1993, Ruzicka Freehand was originally a flowing calligraphy typeface which Ruzicka later developed into a clear italic with just a hint of handwritten style remaining. It is published by Linotype Foundry.

The text of *Vanishing Shoals: a memoir* was typeset in Freight Text. Freight Text is a serif typeface designed by Joshua Darden and published through GarageFonts in 2005. Freight is an extremely versatile superfamily with many different versions available, making it suitable for a wide range of typographic challenges. It is the type family used as part of the identity system for the National Museum of African American History and Culture in Washington D.C.

Vanishing Shoals was designed by Llewellyn Hensley & Content–Aware Graphic Design—**content-aware.design.**

Thank you
for supporting *Unzipped*

Our project is made possible by readers like you. We are infinitely grateful to our patrons who make it possible for us to continue publishing urgent, brave, and true stories! To learn more about supporting us through our subscription program, our online litmag, classes, and workshops, visit **lifein10minutes.com/unzipped.** We would love to write, read, and (metaphorically) unzip with you.

Lightning Source UK Ltd.
Milton Keynes UK
UKHW022111130622
404385UK00014B/269